MEDICINE AND BIOLOGY RESEARCH DEVELOPMENTS

AN ESSENTIAL GUIDE TO MEN'S AND WOMEN'S HEALTH

MEDICINE AND BIOLOGY RESEARCH DEVELOPMENTS

Additional books in this series can be found on Nova's website under the Series tab.

Additional e-books in this series can be found on Nova's website under the eBooks tab.

MEDICINE AND BIOLOGY RESEARCH DEVELOPMENTS

AN ESSENTIAL GUIDE TO MEN'S AND WOMEN'S HEALTH

ALLEN GOODWIN
AND
SHERI LYNCH
EDITORS

nova biomedical
New York

Library of Congress Cataloging-in-Publication Data

ISBN: 978-1-53613-331-8

Published by Nova Science Publishers, Inc. † New York

CONTENTS

PREFACE

An Essential Guide to Men's and Women's Health provides a current summary of bone health in men. Topics include: the epidemiology and temporal trends of low bone mass, osteoporosis and related fractures; the morbidity and mortality associated with osteoporosis and osteoporotic fractures; low bone mass risk factors and etiology; and osteoporotic risk assessment. The book includes a study with the goal of understanding workers' social representation of occupational risks and preventive measures. A qualitative approach was utilised based on social representation theory – processual approach. The sample was comprised of male workers from a municipal service responsible for cleaning and conservation of the public area with no permanent contract in a large city in the South-eastern region of Brazil. The authors describe working conditions and health conditions of men from small enterprises in Campinas' Fruit and Vegetables Warehouse Wholesale. A cross-sectional study with a sample of 200 male workers was developed. Data collection was performed using the following instruments: questionnaire with socio-demographic data, lifestyle, health and work aspects, QSETES elaborated on by author Monteiro and a stress scale adapted by Monteiro based on Elo et al., The authors study the status of women in India, arguing that many poor health outcomes of girls and women can be attributed to their low rank in society. Specifically, the focus is on female economic devaluation, specifically dowry, an issue with historical antecedents that has failed to be addressed or even exacerbated by the entry of the country into the global economy. Postpartum hemorrhage (PPH) is examined as one of the world's leading causes of maternal mortality. Various conservative surgical procedures have been developed in recent years to reduce the need for hysterectomy, including external compression sutures, selective de-vascularization by surgical ligation or radiological embolization of the uterine and pelvic arteries and intrauterine balloon tamponade. The authors also examine the correlation between the development of congenital malformations and teratogenesis brought on by adverse conditions within the *millieur interieur* of the developing embryo, suggesting that the pharmacokinetic processes must be seen in the perspective of maternal and fetal lethal dose parameters. A study on perceived motives for contraceptive interference (CI) is included, hypothesizing that common barriers to male condom use might also be perceived as motives for CI enacted by a man toward his female partner.

Chapter 1 - Although osteoporosis has been viewed as a disease that exclusively affects postmenopausal women, there is growing awareness that osteoporosis and related fractures are a significant public health concern for men worldwide. This chapter will provide a current summary of bone health in men. Topics include: the epidemiology and temporal trends of low bone mass, osteoporosis and related fractures; the morbidity and mortality associated with osteoporosis and osteoporotic fractures; low bone mass risk factors and etiology (including sex hormones); and, osteoporotic risk assessment (bone mineral density T-scores, FRAX, trabecular bone score). An overview of osteoporosis secondary to other conditions and diseases, such as prostate cancer; glucocorticoid therapy, inflammatory conditions, hypogonadism, obesity/T2D, will be included. Finally, the chapter will summarize osteoporosis treatment options for men, including lifestyle modifications (nutrition/exercise) and pharmacotherapy (approved and emerging drugs); clinical trials surrogate endpoints (BMD, bone turnover markers) and fracture-risk reduction. Prevention strategies with an emphasis on physical activity throughout the lifespan will be described.

Chapter 2 - The aim of this study was to understand the worker's social representation of occupational risks and preventive measures. A qualitative approach was utilised, based on social representation theory – processual approach. The sample was composed by male workers, from a municipal service, responsible for cleaning and conservation of the public area with no permanent contract, in a large city of south eastern region Brazil. The research was approved by the Ethical Board. The interviews were recorded and analyzed according to the social theory representation. 43 men answered a semi-structured interview, performed in the workplace, during their working journey. The majority were black (53.5%), 41 years old or over (65.1%) and married (60.5%). Regarding their function, 18 (41.9%) were garbage collectors, 13 (30.2%) were maintenance mechanics, six (14%) were lorry drivers, three (7%) were public area cleaners and three (7%) were vehicles cleaners. The workers speech was analysed and what emerged were the themes of poor working conditions, unsafe workplace environment and unhealthy working conditions. Regarding the occupational risks the authors found: chemical risks (chemical product utilized during the work journey, contact with diesel oil, vehicle painting, the use of thinner, gas, degreaser and powder). Concerning to physical risks the authors found non-ionizing radiation exposure; and the biological risks were the contact with cutting perforating equipment and parts of dead animals. Furthermore, there are other hazards, such as the power relationship among supervisors and the workers, non-compliance with labour legislation and inadequate personal protective equipment. These conditions make these workers subject to situations of occupational vulnerability, requiring measures to improve working conditions and the workplace health promotion. The national and international legislation concerning safety and health at work is not observed and it might lead to unnecessary exposure to chemical and physical agents. Another problem raised by the workers was not having a suitable place for meals during their working journey. The work characteristics, with high physical demand, exposure to cognitive stressors and poor working conditions, might lead to high use of alcohol. The work characteristics indirectly influence the adoption of individual behaviours, which harm their health, increasing the risk of illnesses. The workplace health promotion is essential and occupational health and safety legislation need to be observed, to preserve the health and guarantee a safety and healthy working environment.

Chapter 3 - The aim of this study is to describe working conditions and health conditions of men from micro and small enterprises in Campinas' Fruit and Vegetables Warehouse Wholesale. The warehouse has in the structure small and micro enterprises, with several employment relationships: formal workers, informal workers (freelancers' porters, owners, permission holders, truck drivers, and temporary workers), rural producers and outsourced workers, in four small free markets and four permanent warehouses and small stores. A cross-sectional study with a sample of 200 male workers was developed. Data collection was performed using the following instruments: Questionnaire with Socio-demographic Data, Lifestyle, Health and Work Aspects - QSETS, elaborated by Monteiro. Data were analysed with the program Statistical Analysis Software - SAS® (version 9.1.3, SAS Institute Inc., Cary, NC, USA, 2002-2003). The level of 5% of statistical significance was adopted. Fisher's exact test and Pearson's Chi-square test were applied to assess the associations among variables. All workers were male, the mean age was 36.8 years (SD 12.1), and ranging from 18 to 77 years. 67% of the respondents were married or had a partner and 72% had children. Regarding exposure to risk factors in the workplace, most workers were exposed to repetitive movements (94.5%), stressful work (75%), pace working to finish tasks (65.5%), prolonged bad posture (90%) and weight lifting (96.5%). For chronic diseases, 19% ingested regular medicine; 32.2% reported some health trouble and 19.5% had medical problems. Workers reported body pain in the last week (23.5%) and in the last six months (40.5%). When comparing their health to people at the same age, 46% believed that was similar. Workers with pain reported worse health compared to others at the same age ($p \leq 0.01$). The workers are exposed to poor working conditions, particularly for physical conditions; there is a higher number of chronic smokers and alcohol's consumers when compared with males in national surveys. Their health status is also worse than general male population, especially for those with pain.

Chapter 4 - India's first prime minister, Jawaharlal Nehru, once claimed that one could "tell the condition of a nation by looking at the status of its women." What would Nehru think of India today? Since his reign, there have been great strides in women's achievements, including rising life expectancy and literacy rates. However, despite India's growing role as a global economic powerhouse, the low status of women persists, with enormous consequences for the health of girls and women across their life course. In this chapter, the author argues that many poor health outcomes of girls and women can be attributed to the low status of women in India. The author focuses on female *economic* devaluation, specifically dowry - an issue with historical antecedents that has failed to be addressed and perhaps even exacerbated by the entry of the country into the global economy. Moreover, the failure to consider this bias in the design of population health interventions may be inadvertently contributing to the devaluing of female lives.

Chapter 5 - Postpartum hemorrhage (PPH) continues to be one of the world's leading causes of maternal mortality. Severe PPH has been variously defined as blood loss between 1000mL to 2000 mL or above. Traditionally, peripartum hysterectomy would be performed in patients with massive PPH as a life-saving rescue procedure in those who failed to respond to uterotonics. Various conservative surgical procedures have been developed in recent years to reduce the need for hysterectomy, including external compression sutures, selective de-vascularization by surgical ligation or radiological embolization of the uterine and pelvic arteries and intrauterine balloon tamponade (IUBT). Previously, uterine packing has been employed as a conservative procedure to control PPH by direct pressure effects, but has now been replaced by IUBT. Both uterine specific balloons such as the Bakri balloon, BT- catheter or Belfort-Dildy Obstetrical Tamponade System systems as well as non-uterine specific balloons, such as the Sengstaken- Blakemore tube, Rusch balloons, Foley or condom catheters have also been commonly used, and a high success rate of over 80% in general has been reported. Recent data have shown that increasing use of balloon tamponade was associated with a reduction in the need for more invasive procedures such as radiological uterine artery embolization or compression sutures or for peripartum hysterectomy. The good prognostic factors associated with successful IUBT management include early application of the balloon tamponade in the treatment process and the maintenance of a positive tamponade test, while failed "positive tamponade test", coagulopathy, or placenta accreta are associated with high failure rates. There should be vigilant case selection for using IUBT in severe PPH, and in the presence of adverse risk factors, prompt resort to other treatment modalities, or hysterectomy as a savage procedure.

Chapter 6 - The development of congenital malformations is often associated with teratogenesis brought on by adverse conditions within the *millieur interieur* of the developing embryo. These adverse conditions can range from infective organisms to chemical substances or physical damage exerted onto the developing cells. The teratogenic process is generally considered to give rise to structural abnormalities. The pharmacokinetic processes have to be seen in the perspective of maternal and fetal lethal dose parameters.

Chapter 7 - Contraceptive interference (CI) occurs when a person directly interferes with his or her partner's ability to effectively use contraception before or during sex. Perceived motives for CI warrant empirical study. The authors hypothesized that common barriers to male condom use might also be perceived as motives for CI enacted by a man toward his female partner. In addition, the authors explored potential gender differences in perceptions of these motives. Undergraduates with prior vaginal sex experience (N = 334) read a hypothetical vaginal sex scenario depicting a man's CI behavior. Then participants rated the degree to which they perceived different barriers to male condom use may have motivated the man's behavior. Results showed that all participants perceived that a man's CI behavior was motivated by his intent to enhance his pleasure. Compared to women, men more strongly perceived a man's CI behaviors occurred because the female partner was using another type of birth control, to promote female pleasure, and because the man preferred not to discuss condoms. Compared to men, women more strongly perceived a man's CI behaviors occurred because the female partner was faithful and because the man felt using condoms was difficult. These results suggest that interventions geared toward preventing CI should emphasize that even behaviors apparently motivated by benign intent may yield negative sexual and reproductive health consequences.

In: An Essential Guide … ISBN: 978-1-53613-331-8
Editors: A. Goodwin and S. Lynch

Chapter 1

BONE HEALTH IN MEN: OSTEOPOROSIS UPDATE

Pamela S. Hinton*, PhD
Department of Nutrition and Exercise Physiology,
University of Missouri, Columbia, Missouri, US

ABSTRACT

Although osteoporosis has been viewed as a disease that exclusively affects postmenopausal women, there is growing awareness that osteoporosis and related fractures are a significant public health concern for men worldwide. This chapter will provide a current summary of bone health in men. Topics include: the epidemiology and temporal trends of low bone mass, osteoporosis and related fractures; the morbidity and mortality associated with osteoporosis and osteoporotic fractures; low bone mass risk factors and etiology (including sex hormones); and, osteoporotic risk assessment (bone mineral density T-scores, FRAX, trabecular bone score).

An overview of osteoporosis secondary to other conditions and diseases, such as prostate cancer; glucocorticoid therapy, inflammatory conditions, hypogonadism, obesity/T2D, will be included. Finally, the

* Corresponding Author Email: hintonp@missouri.edu.

chapter will summarize osteoporosis treatment options for men, including lifestyle modifications (nutrition/exercise) and pharmacotherapy (approved and emerging drugs); clinical trials surrogate endpoints (BMD, bone turnover markers) and fracture-risk reduction. Prevention strategies with an emphasis on physical activity throughout the lifespan will be described.

Osteoporosis and Related Fractures Are a Significant Public Health Concern for Men Worldwide

Osteoporosis, a skeletal condition characterized by reduced bone strength and increased risk of low-trauma fractures, affects approximately 200 million people worldwide [1]. Although commonly believed to afflict only postmenopausal women, men also develop osteoporosis and experience osteoporotic fractures. In the United States, 2 million men have osteoporosis and 12 million more have low bone mass [2]. The lifetime risk of osteoporotic fracture in men has been estimated to be between 10% and 25%, depending on the population studied [3, 4], and one in four men over 50 years will experience an osteoporotic fracture in their remaining lifetime [2, 5]. Despite efforts to increase awareness of male osteoporosis [6], the perceptions held by the public and healthcare professionals alike remain grossly inaccurate. Contrary to the prevailing belief that men are at low risk for osteoporosis, men are more likely to suffer an osteoporotic fracture than to develop prostate cancer [1]. Generally, osteoporosis is an under-recognized and under-treated condition, even among individuals who have already experienced a fragility fracture [7]. This is especially true for men who are more likely than women to have undiagnosed or untreated osteoporosis [7, 8]. Even men who, because of another health condition, are under-going treatment known to increase fracture risk are not given adequate medical care [9-11]. Sadly, this lack of appreciation of male osteoporosis contributes to the significantly higher osteoporosis-associated morbidity and mortality in men compared to women. For example, in the first year after hip fracture, one in five men will die, which is nearly double the mortality rate in women [12]. Also contributing to the excess morbidity and mortality in men versus women is the lower adherence to recommendations for primary, secondary, and tertiary prevention [13]. Thus, the misconception that osteoporosis is a "female" disease and the resulting disparities in screening, diagnosis and treatment of osteoporosis exacerbate the magnitude of the public health emergency of male osteoporosis.

PERSONAL AND SOCIETAL COSTS

Osteoporosis and related fractures in men have enormous personal and societal costs, which continue to accumulate after an initial fracture occurs [14]. Individuals who suffer an osteoporotic fracture often experience pain and impaired physical function that results in decreased ability to perform activities of daily living [15]. Consequently, many individuals must move to a assisted-living facility after fracture [16]. Hip fractures are the most devastating fracture, in part because they typically occur later in life than wrist and spine fractures. Wrist fractures usually have only a short-term impact, whereas spine fractures more often result in permanent morbidity [17]. The impairments in physical function and mobility that afflict more than two-thirds of hip fracture patients result in loss of independence. The decrements in physical function have negative psycho-social consequences, including increased depression, isolation, helplessness, and fear of falling. A systematic review of 16 observational studies revealed significantly worse physical and mental health-related quality of life in osteoporotic older men and women with vertebral fracture vs. non-fracture [18]. Individuals who suffer an osteoporotic fracture experience a significant financial burden, which often also impacts their families [15]. After an osteoporotic fracture, individuals may incur out of pocket costs for acute medical care and hospitalization, as well as for long-term medication costs and nursing home care. Furthermore, the family of an individual who suffers a fragility fracture may experience reductions in earnings due to time off work to care for their older family member [19].

The societal burden of osteoporosis includes the direct and indirect costs of osteoporosis-related fractures, the increased health resource utilization associated with such fractures and reduced productivity after fracture. Osteoporosis-related fractures are costly in terms of both the dollar amount and healthcare utilization [20]. Medical and hospital costs associated with osteoporosis-related fractures are significant. Hip fractures incur the greatest cost at both the individual (cost per event) and the aggregate (total cost of all events) levels; however, the costs of vertebral and non-hip, non-vertebral (NHNV) fractures are also considerable [20]. The total cost of fragility fractures in the United States is estimated at $15.8–23.2 billion per year in US dollars, not including indirect costs such as lost productivity of patients and caregivers [9, 15]. Of the cost of fracture treatment, it is estimated that 70% is covered by Medicare, 17% by private insurers, 10% by patients, and the rest by Medicaid [21]. In Europe, the disability due to osteoporosis is greater than that caused by cancers (with the exception of lung cancer) and is similar to or greater than that due to chronic non-communicable diseases, such as rheumatoid arthritis, asthma and high blood pressure related heart disease [22]. Moreover, future costs are expected to increase significantly as the number of osteoporotic fractures grows with the aging population [20]. The 2 million osteoporosis-related fractures reported in 2005 could increase to 3 million by 2025, with annual costs increasing from $16.9 billion to $25.3 billion in US dollars [4]. The costs attributed to osteoporosis-related fractures in men in both Europe and the United States are expected to continue increasing [23-25], and may even exceed those of women [23, 24]. Direct medical costs following fracture account for the largest portion of osteoporosis-related costs in men, and these costs continue to accumulate for at least 1 year following the fracture event. Although women consume a larger portion of total osteoporosis fracture-related costs due to larger numbers of fracture events, the average cost per fracture appears to be higher among men than among women [14].

Epidemiology and Temporal Trends of Low Bone Mass, Osteoporosis and Related Fractures

The prevalence rates of low bone mass, osteoporosis and fragility fractures in men are expected to increase worldwide as the population ages. There are, however, geographic differences in the incidence of osteoporosis and related fractures.

In the United States, 3.4% of men aged 50-59 years have osteoporosis based on femoral neck or lumbar spine bone mineral density (BMD T-score ≤-2.5) and the prevalence of osteoporosis increases to 5.7% in men >65 and 10.9% in men over 80 years of age. Low bone mass (formerly "osteopenia") affects 44% of US men >65 years [26]. As many as one in four men over the age of 50 years will develop at least one osteoporosis-related fracture in their lifetime [2, 22]. In 2005, men accounted for 29% of the 2 million osteoporotic fractures. The lifetime risk of osteoporotic fractures in high-risk Caucasian populations is 20–25% in men [7, 8, 23, 24, 3, 27, 28, 3, 4]. In men, fracture incidence peaks at two times throughout the lifespan [29, 30]. The first peak occurs between 15 and 45 years and is attributed to traumatic fractures of the appendicular skeleton. In this age range, not surprisingly, men are up to 3 times more likely to sustain a fracture than women [29]. The second peak in fracture incidence occurs around 70 years, and is due to low-trauma fractures of the hip, vertebrae, radius, and humerus. In men, the age-related peak in fracture incidence occurs approximately 10 years later than the age-related peak in women.

Worldwide, there is substantial geographic variation in the incidence of hip fracture [31]. Age-adjusted rates of hip fracture in women and men appear highest in Scandinavia and in North America, with almost seven-fold lower rates in Southern Europe [32]. Hip fracture incidence is also lower in Asian and Latin America [33, 34], and rates seem to be lower in rural than in urban areas [35, 36]. The geographical variation in osteoporotic fracture prevalence is similar when fracture incidence in men is examined separately from that of women. Hip fracture rates in men are highest in Northern Europe >150/100,000, followed by North America at 100-150/100,000 and lower rates in Latin America [37]. Regardless of ethnicity, hip fracture risk in men versus women is relatively constant worldwide at a ratio of 1:2 male-to-female [38].

The incidence of osteoporosis and related-fracture is projected to increase significantly as the population ages [39]. Ten million individuals over the age of 50 years in the United States already have osteoporosis, and an additional 34 million individuals have osteopenia [40]. Indeed, the total number of people in the United States with low bone mass could reach 61 million by 2020 [2]. Approximately 1.6 million hip fractures occur worldwide each year. As life expectancy rises around the world, along with the number of elderly individuals in every geographic region, the incidence of hip fractures is estimated to reach 4.5-6.3 million in 2050 [41, 42]. In the United States, the number of individuals aged ≥65 years is expected to reach approximately 72 million in 2030 (corresponding to one in five of the population) [43]. With aging, the incidence of osteoporotic fracture increases in both men and women [4, 39]. Thus, the overall number of fractures is on the rise because the elderly population increases due to the lengthening of the lifespan [44]. However, several studies have shown that the age-specific incidence of major osteoporotic fractures in postmenopausal women, especially hip fracture, has been slightly, but consistently, decreasing for the last 15 years [45-47]. Such trends have been observed in North America, Australia, and several European countries. Although the reason for the plateau or decline in rate of hip fracture in women is not known, changes in later life risk factors, such as physical inactivity or vitamin D insufficiency, are plausible explanations [48]. In contrast to the decline in age-specific fracture incidence in women, the rate of incident hip fracture in men decreased less than in women or even remained stable [47, 49, 50]. In addition, in some European countries and in Japan, age-specific hip fracture incidence continues to increase [51, 52]. Moreover, in much of the world, life expectancy is increasing more for men than for women [53]. Consequently, with greater longevity for men and the increasing growth of the population, the number of men with hip fracture worldwide is estimated to increase markedly in the years to come [41]. Therefore, over the next decades, the number of osteoporotic fractures is expected to increase faster in men than in women. Consequently, fragility fractures in men will constitute higher percentage of all the osteoporotic fractures than they do now.

Morbidity and Mortality Associated with Osteoporosis and Osteoporotic Fractures

Of all osteoporotic fractures in men, hip fractures result in the greatest morbidity and mortality [9]. Each year, about 80,000 men suffer a hip fracture [2]; of these, one in three will die in the first year after a hip fracture and another one-third will fracture again [54]. While the excess risk of death due to hip fractures diminishes with time, there may still be some additional risk for a number of years. For example, approximately 5% of hip fracture patients experience a severe medical complication that increases risk of death [55]. Furthermore, men who suffer a hip fracture have an approximately 2- to 3-fold increased mortality risk relative to women [12]. In addition, the fraction of the potential time of life lost after a hip fracture (taking into account the sex-specific life expectancy) is greater in men than women [44].

Although adverse outcomes are most frequently reported in relation to hip and vertebral fractures, recent data show that NHNV fractures result in significant morbidity and mortality [56]. NHNV fractures are much more numerous and make a larger contribution to the burden of osteoporosis at the population level [57]. In a recent study, of the 952 documented fractures in women and 343 in men, over half were NHNV fractures (486 in women and 173 in men). NHNV fractures were associated with a two-fold relative risk of subsequent fracture in women with even greater risk in men [58]. More importantly, NHNV fractures were associated with 20% excess mortality in the first 5 years after fracture.

Both sex- and gender-based characteristics, i.e., biologic and socio-cultural, respectively [59], influence the pathophysiology, diagnosis, prognosis, and treatment of osteoporosis [60]. These sex and gender differences ultimately influence the rates of morbidity and mortality in men who sustain a hip fracture [8, 61, 62], as men are more likely than women to have osteoporosis that is undiagnosed or undertreated [8, 63, 64]. Likewise, race and ethnicity may influence post-fracture morbidity and mortality. Although data in men are lacking, mortality after hip fracture is higher among African American women than among white women [65, 66]. The factors contributing to the higher mortality rate among African American women after a hip fracture are not completely understood but could reflect their older age at the time of fracture, greater comorbidity, or disparities in health care. Indeed, the average number of diagnoses at admission to the hospital at time of hip fracture is greater among African American women than white women [67]. It is likely that similar racial and ethnic disparities in post-fracture mortality also exist for men.

Risk Factors for Osteoporosis and Related Fractures

Risk factors for osteoporosis and related fractures can be classified as non-modifiable or modifiable. Non-modifiable include sex, race, age, genetics, body mass index, other diseases that impact bone and history of falls. Modifiable risk factors include behavioral risk factors and lifestyle-related diseases [12].

Non-Modifiable Risk Factors

Sex is a strong determinant of fracture risk, and appears to vary with ethnicity and race [68]. In general, white women experience hip fractures about twice the rate of men, especially in countries with high incidence rates; however, the sex difference in hip fracture risk in African Americans and Asians is less than that observed in Caucasian populations. Ethnic and race variability is also lower for men than for women, although white men tend to have slightly higher hip fracture rates than Asian and African American men [31]. The differences in fracture rate is apparently due to differences in body size [69]. Differences in age-related decline in BMD have also been reported, with African American and White men showing similar and greater rates of loss than Asian men [70].

There is increasing evidence for a significant genetic contribution to osteoporosis risk in both men and women [9]. The heritability of BMD, a strong predictor of fracture risk, is 60-80% [71]. A recent study showed that men whose fathers had osteoporosis tended to also have reduced bone size and reduced volumetric BMD [72]. As in women, male offspring of subjects with osteoporosis show reduced bone mass prior to the onset of age-related bone loss [73], suggesting that genetic determinants of osteoporotic risk manifest early in life. Moreover, a recent 3-generation study in men demonstrated that sons of men with osteoporosis have reduced bone size and reduced volumetric BMD, despite normal markers of bone remodeling, consistent with genetic effects on bone being related to skeletal growth rather than age-related decline in bone mass [72]. Interestingly, traumatic fracture prior to older adulthood is associated with low BMD and increased risk of subsequent fracture in older adults of both sexes [74]. Boys who suffer a distal forearm fracture during childhood are at increased risk of subsequent osteoporotic fractures [75]. Current research is focused on identification of genes associated with osteoporosis risk. Multiple genes affect bone development, strength, and density [73, 76].

Other important determinants of fracture risk are factors that increase the likelihood falling [77], as the majority of osteoporotic fractures in men occur after a fall [78]. Other diseases, conditions or their treatment are associated with increased rate of bone loss and/or elevated fracture risk: abdominal aortic calcification [79], decreased thigh subcutaneous fat, and lower appendicular lean mass [80], rheumatoid arthritis [77, 78], Parkinson's Disease [78], Vitamin D insufficiency/deficiency [81, 82], hypogonadism [83, 84], increased sex hormone binding globulin (SHBG) [85], hyperparathyroidism [86], depression [87], stroke [12]. Some of the increased risk is due to poor physical function or increased falls [87, 88]. Individuals with the combination of low D, low estradiol, high SHBG especially at risk [85].

Modifiable Risk Factors

Modifiable risk factors include behavioral risk factors, such as cigarette smoking, excessive alcohol consumption, insufficient or excessive exercise, and lifestyle-related diseases, such as overweight/ obesity and diabetes [12].

Moderate alcohol consumption is associated with higher bone mass [89], and low-to-moderate alcohol use (<27 drinks/week for men and <13 drinks/week for women) has not been associated with any increased fracture risk [90, 91]. The apparent beneficial effects of low or moderate alcohol consumption might be because alcohol slows bone resorption with no effects on bone formation; in turn, the net consequence on mass would be positive [92]. While low or moderate alcohol consumption does seem to negatively affect bone health, excessive and prolonged alcohol consumption lowers bone density and is considered a major risk factor for bone fractures [90, 93].

The prevalence of overweight and obesity in older adults ($BMI \geq 25\, kg/m^2$) is the highest ever reported, and underweight, which is associated with increased risk of osteoporosis, is no longer a problem for most older adults. In the US, 78% of men and 59% of women ≥60 years old are overweight or obese [94]; 34% of women and 37% of men are frankly obese ($BMI \geq 30\, kg/m^2$) [94]. Similar trends are observed in Europe and Australia where the majority of people over 65 years old are overweight or obese [95, 96]. Although the prevalence of obesity is lower in Asian populations, the proportion of overweight older individuals is rapidly increasing [97]. Although previously believed to protect against osteoporosis, excess adiposity is associated with reduced body-weight-adjusted BMD and increased fracture risk [98, 99]. In the Osteoporotic Fractures in Men Study (MrOS), obese men were actually at significantly higher risk for fracture than normal weight men after BMD adjustment [80]. This was particularly obvious with hip fracture: obese men were five-fold more likely to experience a hip fracture than normal weight men when BMD was taken into account. Obese men have slightly higher fracture risk compared with non-obese men, and sarcopenic obesity increases fall and fracture risk in older men [100]. In addition, comorbidities associated with overweight and obesity, such as type 2 diabetes [101], abdominal obesity [102], insulin resistance [103], hyperglycemia [104] and dyslipidemia [105] might contribute to the detrimental changes in bone's structural and material properties [106-109]. Hypercholesterolemia is associated with reduced osteoblastogenesis and osteoblast formation and with increased osteoclastogenesis [106-109]. Insulin resistance of bone is associated with reduce bone formation and deleterious changes in trabecular micro-architecture [110], while whole body insulin resistance and hyperglycemia facilitate accumulation of advanced glycation end-products (AGEs) in bone [111, 112]. Modifiable risk factors should be targets of behavior-change interventions, including smoking cessation, moderation of alcohol intake, increase physical activity, and reduction in fall risk [113]. Very few studies have examined the efficacy of such intervention to increase BMD or reduce fracture risk. Smoking cessation in men reduces fracture incidence in men who were former smokers relative to men who continued to smoke [114, 115]. On the other hand, reduction in alcohol intake from heavy intake to light alcohol consumption did not significantly impact fracture risk in one study [116]. However, considering the other deleterious effects associated with excessive alcohol intake, counseling men with heavy alcohol consumption on the potential general health benefits associated with reduced alcohol intake is warranted. A very recent analysis of the MrOS data revealed that older age (>75 years), low BMD, smoking, greater height and height loss since age 25 years, history of fracture, use of tricyclic antidepressants, history of myocardial infarction, hyperthyroidism or Parkinson's disease, lower protein intake, and lower executive function were all independently associated with a higher risk of hip fracture [80]. Hip fracture risk was increased by a stunning 50-fold in men with osteoporosis based on BMD who also had at least four of the above risk factors. From a practical perspective, assessment of these risk factors could readily be included in routine clinical care of older men to identify patients at very high risk of fracture [80].

Etiology of Age-Related Osteoporosis

Increased bone fragility can be attributed to changes in bone's structural and material properties at all levels of bone's hierarchical structure from the whole bone to ultrastructure of collagen/mineral crystals [117]. Thus, BMD, which predicts fracture risk at the population level, is just one determinant of bone's fracture resistance [118]. As fracture risk increases at age ~70 years, in association with accelerated bone loss in men, examination of age-related changes in bone is relevant to understanding fracture risk.

Sex Differences in Cortical and Cancellous Bone Mass and Structure throughout the Lifespan

Consistent with their larger body size, men have 35–42% larger bone areas (depending on the specific skeletal site examined) than women in young adulthood (age range 20–29 years) [119]. In both sexes, bone area increases during adulthood by ~15%, indicative of ongoing periosteal bone growth. However, the increase in bone size, which results in greater whole-bone strength, is offset by marked decreases in volumetric BMD (vBMD). Cancellous vBMD begins to decline in young adulthood, with ongoing cancellous bone loss continuing throughout the lifespan. Cortical bone mass is maintained until middle age when sex steroids decline, abruptly in women and gradually in men, contributing to cortical bone loss [29, 120]. Decreases in vBMD in both cancellous and cortical bone are greater in women than in men, due to the combined effect of menopause and subsequent loss of estrogen and aging. While the decline in cancellous bone volume fraction (BV/TV) is similar between women and men, there are notable differences in trabecular microarchitecture. Women exhibit a loss of trabeculae (Tb.N), while men show a decrease in trabecular thickness (Tb.Th) with preservation of Tb.N. This difference contributes to the sex difference in fragility fracture rate, as the loss of trabeculae is much more detrimental to biomechanical properties than an equivalent decline in Tb.Th [121]. Aging is associated with greater loss of cortical bone than of cancellous bone, as well as with marked increases in cortical porosity [122] due to bone resorption on endocortical surfaces. It is important to note that these detrimental changes in trabecular and cortical microarchitecture cannot be detected by dual-energy X-ray absorptiometry (DXA) [29] and, as such, cannot be used clinically as indicators of fracture risk.

Hormone-Mediated Changes in Bone Formation and Resorption

Ultimately, the changes in cancellous and cortical bone mass and structure are determined by the balance between bone formation and bone resorption in the remodeling process. Both the balance and coupling of bone resorption and formation depend on the number and activity of osteoclasts and osteoblasts, as well as their coordination by osteocytes [123]. An increase in osteoclast number or activity relative to the need for remodeling or insufficient osteoblast number or formation relative to the need for resorption cavity refilling are responsible for the pathophysiological changes of metabolic bone diseases [124, 125], including postmenopausal and age-related bone loss. Hormonal changes associated with aging play an important role in the etiology of age-related bone loss in men. Most of the structural abnormalities in cancellous and cortical bone of men with osteoporosis are related to altered endocrine function, particularly to impaired insulin-like growth factor-I (IGF-I) and sex hormone action [30, 126-129].

Sex Steroids

Men do not experience a dramatic loss of androgens analogous to the abrupt decline in estrogens at menopause. Rather, serum androgen and estrogen levels decline slowly, but progressively starting at 50-60 years of age [130]. Because sex hormone binding globulin (SHBG) increases with aging, the free bioavailable fractions of estrogens and androgens are disproportionately affected [126]. Estrogens and androgens slow the rate of bone remodeling and maintain balance between bone resorption and formation by controlling the differentiation and proliferation of both osteoclasts and osteoblasts [123]. In addition, sex steroids influence the lifespan of both of these cells in opposite direction by exerting pro-apoptotic effects on osteoclasts and anti-apoptotic effects on mature osteoblasts and osteocytes [131-133]. Estrogen or androgen deficiency causes loss of bone mass that results from increased osteoclast and osteoblast numbers, and increased resorption and formation, albeit unbalanced [124].

It remains unclear whether the decrease in testosterone that occurs with aging is the direct cause of aging-associated bone loss. Several studies have shown that serum estradiol levels are more robustly associated with BMD in older men [134]. Testosterone is aromatized to estradiol in men, and, in fact, the major source of circulating estradiol in men is aromatization of testosterone. It appears the primary role of androgen aromatization into estrogens in the regulation of bone homeostasis in adult men [135-137]. However, there are androgen receptors on bone cells [138], and androgens might stimulate periosteal apposition in cortical bone. The decline in androgens with age may have indirect skeletal effects. Androgen-deficiency-induced loss of muscle mass likely leads to decreased lower body strength, decreased mechanical loading by muscle contraction forces, and increased propensity to fall [126].

IGF-I

IGF-I has both endocrine and paracrine activity [139]. Circulating IGF-I is thought to be derived from hepatic production under the control of growth hormone. IGF-I produced by pre-osteoblasts, mature osteoblasts, osteocytes, osteoclasts, and skeletal muscle cells acts in a paracrine fashion

[139]. The contribution of endocrine versus paracrine IGF-I to bone modeling and remodeling remains an active area of research. The age-related decline in skeletal IGF-I suggests that IGF available might be insufficient for new bone formation and highlights the importance of adequate IGF-I deposition into the skeleton during modeling and remodeling [140].

Numerous cross-sectional studies in clinical populations have demonstrated an inverse association between circulating IGF-I and bone mass [139]. Patients with osteoporosis have reduced serum IGF-I, which is an independent predictor of osteoporosis and related fractures [140]. Likewise, bone marrow IGF-I concentrations are 40% lower in people with osteoporosis compared to age-matched controls [141]. Skeletal IGF-I content in human bone declines almost 60% between 20 and 60 years of age [142] and correlates even more strongly with bone volume than serum IGF-1 [140, 143]. Men with low serum IGF-1 have an increased risk of hip and vertebral fractures, two of the most clinically important fractures. The association between serum IGF-1 and incident fracture risk in older men is partly mediated by BMD [144].

Osteoporotic Fracture Risk Assessment

Bone Mineral Density

The identification of men at high risk of fracture is inadequate, in part, because there is a lack of standard BMD-screening protocol for men [26]. Physicians are less likely to recommend osteoporosis screening, including dual-energy X-ray absorptiometry, for their male patients [145]. Increasing age, history of fragility fracture, and low bone mineral density (BMD) measured by dual energy X-ray absorptiometry (DXA) are important risk factors of fracture [44]. In MrOS, each SD in T-score below the mean was associated with a 3-fold increase in fracture risk [146]. Nevertheless, only 20% of men who sustain a hip fracture or major osteoporotic fracture have osteoporosis diagnosed by DXA, which is one-half as many compared with women [39, 88, 147]. The National Osteoporosis Foundation, Endocrine Society, International Society Clinical Densitometry recommend screening for all men over age 70 years and for men 50-70 years with one or more risk factor [148]. Screening is also recommended for men prescribed long-term glucocorticoids, HIV medications, androgen-deprivation therapy, or with hypogonadism, primary hyperparathyroidism, or intestinal disorders [148].

FRAX

While BMD is a predictor of future fracture, many fractures occur in individuals with normal BMD [118]. To improve identification of individuals at risk for future fracture, the World Health Organization developed the Fracture Risk Assessment Tool (FRAX). The FRAX algorithm integrates clinical risk factors and femoral neck BMD to estimate the 10-yr probability of a hip or major osteoporotic (clinical spine, forearm, hip, or shoulder) fracture in men and women [149]. Clinical risk factors included in the FRAX model include: age, gender, weight, height, a personal history of previous fragility fracture, history of parental hip fracture, current smoking, glucocorticoid use, rheumatoid arthritis diagnosis, alcohol intake of greater than three units per day, a known disorder strongly associated with secondary osteoporosis, femoral neck BMD, or T-score. Another algorithm for fracture risk prediction is the Garvan nomogram [150]. It takes into account history of fractures and that of falls. Falls, especially multiple falls, seem to be associated with a substantial increase in the risk of peripheral fracture in the elderly men [151]. Both FRAX and the Garvan nomogram have been introduced only recently and few studies assessed their utility in men [152].

Another important consideration in the screening of men for osteoporotic fracture risk is men's attitudes towards osteoporosis screening. There are striking sex differences in perspectives, beliefs, and behaviors, with women readily accepting and undergoing regular osteoporosis screening and being more likely to take nutritional supplements than men. In contrast, men do not view osteoporosis screening as necessary, and, in one study, the majority would reject screening, despite almost half of respondents having sustained a prior fracture [145].

Osteoporosis Secondary to Other Conditions and Diseases

Osteoporosis is categorized as primary or secondary depending on the etiology. Age-related and idiopathic osteoporosis is considered primary osteoporosis, while that associated from lifestyle behaviors, comorbid conditions or medical treatment is considered secondary osteoporosis.

Male osteoporosis that can be linked to or explained by causes other than aging is generally classified as secondary male osteoporosis. Chronic diseases associated with secondary osteoporosis include: chronic obstructive pulmonary disease (COPD) [153, 154], cardiovascular disease [155], rheumatoid arthritis [156], osteoarthritis [157], and multiple sclerosis [158], chronic kidney or liver disease, primary hyper-parathyroidism, inflammatory bowel disease; Celiac disease, Crohn's disease, prostate cancer [9]. The increased risk associated with these diseases is due to endocrine changes, chronic inflammatory state and/or decreased nutrient absorption [159]. Medications that are associated with increased fracture risk include: antiepileptic medications, thyroxine over-replacement, human immunodeficiency virus and/or its treatment with protease inhibitors, immunosuppressive medications, and androgen-deprivation therapy [160].

The three most common causes of secondary osteoporosis in men, which account for up to 40% of all men with osteoporosis, are alcohol abuse, glucocorticoid excess (most commonly from chronic glucocorticoid therapy), and hypogonadism [126]. Despite the higher prevalence of osteoporosis, osteopenia, and fractures in patients with these characteristics, testing and treatment rates are low [9]. Men at clear risk for osteoporotic fracture, such as those who have already suffered a fragility fracture, those who are on oral glucocorticoids, and those on androgen-deprivation therapy for prostate cancer are not evaluated and/or treated for osteoporosis. Specifically, in studies of secondary fracture prevention, men are less likely than women to have evaluation or treatment of osteoporosis [11]. Men at risk for glucocorticoid-induced osteoporosis are also less likely to be evaluated and/or treated [161]. Most men on androgen-deprivation therapy for prostate cancer have little attention paid to their osteoporosis risk, despite the fact that the fracture rate may be as high as 20% in the first 5 years of androgen-deprivation therapy [10, 162].

TREATMENT OF OSTEOPOROSIS IN MEN

The overriding treatment goal in the management of osteoporosis is the prevention of future fractures [163]. Men at significantly increased risk for fracture are those who have already suffered a fracture. A history of osteoporotic fracture is associated with a two- to four-fold higher risk of another osteoporotic fracture [44, 151, 164]. However, while 50 percent of women who sustain a fragility fracture benefit from bone densitometry and/or anti-osteoporotic treatment [7, 8], less than 10 percent of men who sustained an osteoporotic fracture will have bone densitometry and/or osteoporotic treatment [7, 8]. In some studies, only 1 out of 20 men having sustained a hip fracture (and were hospitalized for this fracture) benefited from bone densitometry and/or anti-osteoporotic treatment [8]. Even men receiving chronic glucocorticoid therapy or androgen-deprivation therapy are not systematically screened and treated for osteoporosis [165, 166]. As with screening, universal guidelines for treatment of osteoporosis in men are lacking, which might contribute to the low rates of treatment in men.

The National Osteoporosis Foundation [167] and the Endocrine Society [168] endorse similar treatment recommendations. Treatment is recommended for men with a non-traumatic hip or vertebral fracture; BMD T-score <-2.5 for femoral neck total hip or lumbar spine; BMD T-score between -1.0 and -2.5 and a 10-year probability of hip fracture ≥3% or a 10-year probability of a major fracture ≥20% based on the US-adapted

FRAX. The Endocrine Society also recommends treatment for me >50 years old on long-term glucocorticoid therapy [168].

Non-Pharmacologic Treatment: Modifiable Risk Factors

Non-pharmacologic treatment should focus on modifiable risk factors, including increased physical activity, avoidance of smoking and excess alcohol intake, a total calcium intake of 1000 to 1500 mg per day and a total vitamin D intake of 600 to 800 IU per day [169]. The efficacy of calcium and vitamin D treatment for fracture prevention in osteoporotic women is controversial [170]. Meta-analyses of several large trials of both calcium and vitamin D supplementation have shown a small reduction in fracture risk, particularly among the institutionalized elderly or those with a low intake of calcium or vitamin D [171]. Supplementation with vitamin D alone does not reduce fracture risk or increase BMD, although daily supplementation might reduce the risk of falls [172]. However, high doses of vitamin D (i.e., those that producing 25-hydroxyvitamin D levels >100 nmol/L) appear to increase fracture rates [173, 174]. Interestingly, similar adverse effects of high doses of vitamin D on falls risk have recently been reported [173, 175, 176]. Thus, in osteoporosis management, ensuring that patients are not vitamin D deficient is sensible, and this can be assured in those at risk with a daily supplement of 400–800 units. Likewise, ensuring adequate calcium intake through diet or supplements is also prudent; the recommendation for men 50-70 y is 100 mg/d and >70 y is 1200 mg/d [177].

Drug Therapy

Pharmacologic treatment of male osteoporosis limited by: 1) lack of drug efficacy data in men despite abundance of such data in women; 2) inadequate knowledge of healthcare providers; and, 3) poor treatment compliance and adherence. Despite the wealth of available data from numerous studies in women, the current strategy of drug development for the treatment of osteoporosis in men is such that there is a delay of several years before clinical trial data in men become available. From a pragmatic point of view, it is unlikely that drugs for the specific treatment of osteoporosis in men will be developed [44]. Sex-specific differences in the development of bone exist [178] and may have consequences on the later pathophysiologic process of osteoporosis in men and women [60]. Pharmacologic agents for the treatment of osteoporosis can be classified as either anti-resorptive (i.e., targeting osteoclast-mediated bone resorption) or anabolic (i.e., stimulating osteoblasts to form new bone) [169]. Drugs to treat men with osteoporosis include the anti-resorptive bisphosphonates and denosumab and teriparatide, the only anabolic agent approved for human use in the US, parathyroid hormone, which is approved for use in Europe [179]. Randomized, placebo-controlled studies examining the efficacy of osteoporosis medications in men are rare, and the majority of such existing studies used surrogate end-points, such as BMD or bone turnover markers, rather than fracture [148].

Bisphosphonates increase BMD by inhibiting bone remodeling. Oral and intravenous bisphosphonates are available, and, as a class, the bisphosphonates are the most commonly prescribed drug for osteoporosis treatment [169]. In women, either oral or intravenous bisphosphonates reduce the risk of fractures [180, 181]. Although data in men are limited, bisphosphonates also appear to increase BMD and to reduce bone resorption and fracture risk. In a 2-year study of 1200 men, the intravenous bisphosphonate zoledronic acid resulted in fewer morphological vertebral fractures compared to placebo infusion [182]. In another trial involving women and men who were randomly assigned to receive zoledronic acid or placebo within 90 days after surgical repair of a hip fracture, those who received zoledronic acid had a significantly lower rate of subsequent clinical fractures (by 35%) [183]. Two rare, but serious, adverse effects have been reported: atypical femoral fractures [184], and osteonecrosis of the jaw [185].

The other anti-resorptive drug available is denosumab, which is a monoclonal antibody to RANKL that reduces bone resorption by inhibiting osteoclast differentiation and activity. The drug is administered as a subcutaneous injection once every six months. Denosumab was the first biologic approved for treatment of osteoporosis and specifically osteoporosis in men [186]. Denosumab is also recommended for men with non-metastatic prostate cancer on androgen-deprivation therapy [187]. Men with low BMD show increases BMD of the lumbar spine after denosumab treatment [188]. In men on androgen-deprivation therapy for prostate cancer, denosumab resulted in fewer morphological vertebral fractures compared to placebo [189]. In one study, denosumab was associated with lower costs and higher health benefits than zoledronic acid in elderly men with osteoporosis [187].

Teriparatide, which the first 34 amino acids of parathyroid hormone, is the only anabolic agent for osteoporosis available in the United States. Full-length parathyroid hormone is approved for use in Europe. Chronically elevated parathyroid hormone, such as occurs in hyperparathyroidism, causes bone loss. However, intermittent administration of teriparatide given as a once daily subcutaneous bolus injection activates osteoblast [190] and increases bone formation. In women, teriparatide treatment results in fewer fractures [191], and teriparatide produces similar changes in BMD and bone turnover markers in men and women [191, 192]. Teriparatide treatment resulted in fewer vertebral fractures in men and women with glucocorticoid-induced osteoporosis, compared to those treated with the bisphosphonate alendronate [193]. Teriparatide is administered by daily self-injection and is approved for up to 2 years of use [169].

Bisphosphonate Drug Holidays

The increased risk of atypical femur fractures with long-term bisphosphonate treatment [184, 194], had led to recommended drug holidays (i.e., temporary discontinuation for up to 5 years). The optimal duration of a drug holiday has not been determined [195]. Two randomized trials showed that when alendronate was discontinued after 5 years, skeletal benefits (BMD and bone turnover markers) were maintained for up to 5 years. Similar results were seen following cessation of zoledronic acid after 3 years of use [196, 197]. The current recommendation is for drug holidays in patients who are at lower fracture risk, based on hip BMD and vertebral-fracture status at the time of potential discontinuation [198, 199] and that treatment generally be reinitiated after no longer than 5 years. The duration of the action of bisphosphonate varies between drugs, and the length of a drug holiday should reflect these differences. A 6-month holiday is adequate for the anti-resorptive effects of risedronate to resolve, while alendronate holidays of 1–2 years are used, and the duration of the action of zoledronate is even longer [200]. There is no cure for osteoporosis. Consequently, physicians and patients should recognize that life-long treatment is needed and that drug therapy will be reinitiated after a drug holiday. The alternative is that drug holidays might be too long and fractures that could have been prevented might occur [200].

Treatment Sequence

Both anabolic and potent anti-resorptive agents (bisphosphonates, denosumab) improve bone mineral density (BMD) and reduce risk of fracture in patients who have not been on prior osteoporosis treatments [183, 191, 201-203]. However, the effects of most osteoporosis medications are significantly different in patients who have already been treated with another osteoporosis drug [204-206]. Data suggest that patients who are treatment-naïve should be treated with an anabolic therapy first, followed by anti-resorptive therapy [207]. The common clinical practice of first treating patients with an anti-resorptive drug first, and then switching them to teriparatide only if they do not show an adequate response to the anti-resorptive or suffer a fracture does not optimize the benefits of anabolic treatment [208].

Emerging and Other Drug Therapies

Drugs currently in clinical trials include the anabolic PTHrP and the anti-resorptive odanacatib, which is a monoclonal antibody to cathepsin K. Blosozumab, an antibody to sclerostin the Wnt-signaling antagonist, increased bone formation in Phase II clinical trials [209].

Testosterone replacement therapy increases BMD in hypogonadal men with osteoporosis [210] with a greater effect in cancellous bone and in the spine versus hip [211]. However, the safety of testosterone replacement therapy has recently come under scrutiny because of increased cardio-vascular morbidity associated with exogenous testosterone administration. The FDA issued a safety warning that testosterone replacement therapy should not be used to treat aging alone [212].

Inadequate Knowledge about Osteoporosis among Physicians and Patients

Surveys of healthcare providers involved in the treatment of osteoporosis patients suggest that they have inadequate knowledge about osteoporosis management and prevention [213]. Only 50% of physicians report that their knowledge is adequate and that they are familiar with most recent osteoporosis treatment guidelines [214, 215]. Family medicine specialists reportedly have greater knowledge of osteoporosis diagnosis and treatment than general practitioners [216]. Women physicians are more knowledgeable [215, 217, 218], an observation explained by an overall greater awareness of women about osteoporosis. Younger physicians [216, 217] and those with less seniority [216] have also been reported to have greater knowledge about osteoporosis. Physicians report that the primary barriers to optimal treatment are lack of consistent compliance on the part of patients and lack of knowledge on the part of physicians. In the United States, direct pharmaceutical advertising to patients is legal, and there are many advertisements for medications for erectile dysfunction or hypo-gonadism. In contrast, all osteoporosis medication advertisements are directed to postmenopausal women. Thus, both patients and clinicians have less concern about osteoporosis in men, compared to women, even though the mortality after hip fracture is twice as high in men as it is in women [219, 220].

Treatment Adherence

In a recent systematic review, Mikyas reported that one-third to two-thirds of men were non-adherent to bisphosphonate treatment for osteoporosis and, as expected, non-adherence was associated with worse clinical outcomes [14]. A retrospective chart review study reported similar rates of non-adherence over two years [13]. Poor compliance was more likely in prescription of the first anti-osteoporotic regimen by an orthopedist. Men with rheumatoid arthritis or who had undergone BMD measurement before therapy had a lower risk of non-adherence. Knowledge and beliefs about osteoporosis may interact with gender and race to impact adherence. The majority of the men have limited understanding of osteoporosis disease process, prevention, and risk factors [221]. Men have even less knowledge about the relationship between osteoporosis and men's health than between osteoporosis and women's health [222, 223]. The limited knowledge displayed by men about osteoporosis spans international lines [221].

Men with osteoporosis may seek healthcare only as a last resort because of the importance of maintaining a hegemonic masculine identity by being physically active and strong, and engaging in usual activities, traditional gender roles, and occupations [224]. Osteoporosis often challenges these roles, and men report feeling feminized by osteoporosis and its frequent attribution as a "female disease" [225]. Race and ethnicity may also impact treatment adherence. Black Americans were less likely to express a willingness to have fracture surgery compared to White Americans [226]. Black Americans also reported greater levels of healthcare distrust, lower education levels, greater comorbidities, and fewer prior surgeries compared to White Americans. Black patients also have greater distrust of physicians, particularly distrust of primary care physicians' knowledge and engagement in bone health, and medications [227-230].

Prevention Strategies with an Emphasis on Diet and Physical Activity

Diet

The importance of adequate calcium and vitamin D intake to bone health is well known. However, there is evidence from large population-based studies that habitual, regular intake of certain foods is associated with reduced fracture risk. Specifically, a Mediterranean diet that emphasizes fruits, vegetables, fish, whole grains and monounsaturated fats, and alcohol in moderation is associated with skeletal health and fracture risk [231, 232, 233, 234, 235]. In addition, low protein intake (i.e., <11% of total energy intake) in men was associated with increased fracture risk [236]. Taken together, these recent studies support the consumption of a Mediterranean diet and adequate dietary to improve bone health [237].

Physical Activity

The American College of Sports Medicine recommends weight-bearing endurance activities, including those that involve jumping (such as tennis) and jogging, three to five times per week and resistance exercise two to three times per week to preserve bone health during adulthood [238]. Resistance training is recommended by the National Strength and Conditioning Association to increase bone mineral density (BMD) or to prevent age-associated reductions in BMD [239]. The Surgeon General's Report on Bone Health also recommends progressive resistance training, as well as daily jump-training and participation in weight-bearing recreational activities, for individuals who can tolerate high-impact activity [40].

Although physical activity during growth appears to have beneficial effects on bone that persist into adulthood, activity-associated bone loading after skeletal growth is complete is also important for bone health during middle-age and older adulthood [240]. Bone-loading during adolescence and young adulthood were significant, positive predictors of BMD of the whole body, total hip, and lumbar spine, adjusting for lean body mass and/or age in the regression models. Men who participate in a high-impact activity as adults have greater lumbar spine BMD than men who do not participate in high-impact activity [241]. Moreover, men who participate in a high-impact activity throughout their life have greater hip and lumbar spine BMD than non-participants [241]. In addition to increasing BMD, bone loading during adulthood increases bone size, cortical area, and strength [242] and reduces fracture risk [243, 244]. Even in much older men (~80 years) current physical activity positively affects bone, in part by reducing endosteal expansion, that is, bone loss [245].

Most human data that compare activities that differ in impact magnitude are cross-sectional studies of participants in various sports or leisure time activities. Randomized longitudinal studies that evaluate the effects of exercise or compare the effect of different types of exercise on bone mass in men are limited. In a randomized high-impact, unilateral exercise intervention, high-impact exercise (jumping) increased femoral neck BMD in 70-year-old men [246]. Similarly, 18 months of resistance training combined with jumping exercises led to significantly improved femoral neck BMD and lumbar spine trabecular BMD in men aged 50 to 79 years [247]. In a 12-month, randomized intervention, resistance training or jump training increased lumbar spine BMD [248] and resistance training increased total hip BMD in men with low bone mass. Changes in BMD were accompanied by decreased serum markers of bone resorption and increased bone formation. Circulating sclerostin, which antagonizes Wnt signaling and bone formation, was decreased and IGF-I increased after 12 months of resistance training or jump training [249]. It appears that resistance training alone or in combination with impact-loading activities are most osteogenic for this population, whereas the walking trials had limited effect on BMD. Therefore, regular resistance training and impact-loading activities should be considered as a strategy to prevent osteoporosis in middle-aged and older men [250]. Of note, physicians who treat patients with osteoporosis appear unaware of the benefits of exercise for individuals with low bone mass [251], suggesting an opportunity for physician education.

CONCLUSION

Osteoporosis is growing public health concern as the population ages. This is especially true for men who are much more likely to be undiagnosed and untreated, even after an osteoporotic fracture. There is an urgent need for education of healthcare providers and patients regarding osteoporosis in men to increase awareness and overcome gender-based disparities in diagnosis, treatment and prognosis.

REFERENCES

[1] International Osteoporosis Foundation. *Osteoporosis Facts and Statistics*. Available from: https://www.iofbonehealth.org/references-facts-and-statistics.

[2] *National Osteoporosis Foundation*. Available from: https://www.nof.org/.

[3] Nguyen ND, Ahlborg HG, Center JR, Eisman JA and Nguyen TV. Residual lifetime risk of fractures in women and men. *J Bone Miner Res* 2007;22:781-8.

[4] Burge R, Dawson-Hughes B, Solomon DH, Wong JB, King A and Tosteson A. Incidence and economic burden of osteoporosis-related fractures in the United States, 2005-2025. *J Bone Miner Res* 2007;22:465-75.

[5] Center for Disease Control and Prevention. Falls among older adults: An overview. 2013; Available from: http://www.cdc.gov/home andrecreational men: a review. *Bone Res* 2014;2:14001.
[6] Panneman MJ, Lips P, Sen SS and Herings RM. Under treatment with anti-osteoporotic drugs after hospitalization for fracture. *Osteoporos Int* 2004;15:120-4.
[7] Kiebzak GM, Beinart GA, Perser K, Ambrose CG, Siff SJ and Heggeness MH. Under treatment of osteoporosis in men with hip fracture. *Arch Intern Med* 2002;162:2217-22.
[8] Willson T, Nelson SD, Newbold J, Nelson RE and LaFleur J. The clinical epidemiology of male osteoporosis: a review of the recent literature. *Clin Epidemiol* 2015;7:65-76.
[9] Shahinian VB, Kuo YF, Freeman JL and Goodwin JS. Risk of fracture after androgen deprivation for prostate cancer. *N Engl J Med* 2005;352:154-64.
[10] Jennings LA, Auerbach AD, Maselli J, Pekow PS, Lindenauer PK and Lee SJ. Missed opportunities for osteoporosis treatment in patients hospitalized for hip fracture. *J Am Geriatr Soc* 2010;58:650-7.
[11] Drake MT and Khosla S. Male osteoporosis. *Endocrinol Metab Clin North Am* 2012;41:629-41.
[12] Chiu CK, Kuo MC, Yu SF, Su BY and Cheng TT. Adherence to osteoporosis regimens among men and analysis of risk factors of poor compliance: a 2-year analytical review. *BMC Musculoskelet Disord* 2013;14:276.
[13] Mikyas Y, Agodoa I and Yurgin N. A systematic review of osteoporosis medication adherence and osteoporosis-related fracture costs in men. *Appl Health Econ Health Policy* 2014;12:267-77.
[14] United States Office of the Surgeon General. *Bone Health and Osteoporosis: A Report of the Surgeon General.* 5, "The Burden of Bone Disease." 2004; Available from: https://www.ncbi.nlm.nih.gov/books/NBK45502/.
[15] Salkeld G, Cameron ID, Cumming RG, Easter S, Seymour J, Kurrle SE and Quine S. Quality of life related to fear of falling and hip

fracture in older women: a time trade off study. *BMJ* 2000;320:341-6.

[16] Kanis JA and Johnell O. The burden of osteoporosis. *J Endocrinol Invest* 1999;22:583-8.

[17] Al-Sari UA, Tobias J and Clark E. Health-related quality of life in older people with osteoporotic vertebral fractures: a systematic review and meta-analysis. *Osteoporos Int* 2016;27:2891-900.

[18] Brainsky A, Glick H, Lydick E, Epstein R, Fox KM, Hawkes W, Kashner TM, Zimmerman SI and Magaziner J. The economic cost of hip fractures in community-dwelling older adults: a prospective study. *J Am Geriatr Soc* 1997;45:281-7.

[19] Budhia S, Mikyas Y, Tang M and Badamgarav E. Osteoporotic fractures: a systematic review of U.S. healthcare costs and resource utilization. *Pharmacoeconomics* 2012;30:147-70.

[20] Blume SW and Curtis JR. Medical costs of osteoporosis in the elderly Medicare population. *Osteoporos Int* 2011;22:1835-44.

[21] Johnell O and Kanis JA. An estimate of the worldwide prevalence and disability associated with osteoporotic fractures. *Osteoporos Int* 2006;17:1726-33.

[22] Konnopka A, Jerusel N and Konig HH. The health and economic consequences of osteopenia- and osteoporosis-attributable hip fractures in Germany: estimation for 2002 and projection until 2050. *Osteoporos Int* 2009;20:1117-29.

[23] King AB, Tosteson AN, Wong JB, Solomon DH, Burge RT and Dawson-Hughes B. Interstate variation in the burden of fragility fractures. *J Bone Miner Res* 2009;24:681-92.

[24] Burge RT, King AB, Balda E and Worley D. Methodology for estimating current and future burden of osteoporosis in state populations: application to Florida in 2000 through 2025. *Value Health* 2003;6:574-83.

[25] Gourlay ML, Overman RA and Ensrud KE. Bone Density Screening and Re-screening in Postmenopausal Women and Older Men. *Curr Osteoporos Rep* 2015;13:390-8.

[26] *Osteoporosis in Men: The Effects of Gender on Skeletal Health.* 2010, London: Elsevier.

[27] Lippuner K, Johansson H, Kanis JA and Rizzoli R. Remaining lifetime and absolute 10-year probabilities of osteoporotic fracture in Swiss men and women. *Osteoporos Int* 2009;20:1131-40.

[28] Khosla S, Amin S and Orwoll E. Osteoporosis in men. *Endocr Rev* 2008;29:441-64.

[29] Gielen E, Vanderschueren D, Callewaert F and Boonen S. Osteoporosis in men. *Best Pract Res Clin Endocrinol Metab* 2011;25:321-35.

[30] Cummings SR and Melton LJ. Epidemiology and outcomes of osteoporotic fractures. *Lancet* 2002;359:1761-7.

[31] Johnell O, Gullberg B, Allander E and Kanis JA. The apparent incidence of hip fracture in Europe: a study of national register sources. *Osteoporos Int* 1992;2:298-302.

[32] Yan L, Zhou B, Prentice A, Wang X and Golden MH. Epidemiological study of hip fracture in Shenyang, People's Republic of China. *Bone* 1999;24:151-5.

[33] Morales-Torres J and Gutierrez-Urena S. The burden of osteoporosis in Latin America. *Osteoporos Int* 2004;15:625-32.

[34] Kaastad TS, Meyer HE and Falch JA. Incidence of hip fracture in Oslo, Norway: differences within the city. *Bone* 1998;22:175-8.

[35] Sanders KM, Nicholson GC, Ugoni AM, Seeman E, Pasco JA and Kotowicz MA. Fracture rates lower in rural than urban communities: the Geelong Osteoporosis Study. *J Epidemiol Community Health* 2002;56:466-70.

[36] International Osteoporosis Foundation. *Osteoporosis Epidemiology.* 2015 [cited 2017; Available from: https://www.iofbonehealth.org/epidemiology.

[37] Kanis JA, Oden A, McCloskey EV, Johansson H, Wahl DA and Cooper C. A systematic review of hip fracture incidence and probability of fracture worldwide. *Osteoporos Int* 2012;23:2239-56.

[38] Schuit SC, van der Klift M, Weel AE, de Laet CE, Burger H, Seeman E, Hofman A, Uitterlinden AG, van Leeuwen JP and Pols HA.

Fracture incidence and association with bone mineral density in elderly men and women: the Rotterdam Study. *Bone* 2004;34:195-202.

[39] United States Department of Health and Human Services. *Bone Health and Osteoporosis: A Report of the Surgeon General,* 2004: Rockville, MD.

[40] Gullberg B, Johnell O and Kanis JA. World-wide projections for hip fracture. *Osteoporos Int* 1997;7:407-13.

[41] Cooper C and Melton LJ, 3rd. Epidemiology of osteoporosis. *Trends Endocrinol Metab* 1992;3:224-9.

[42] Center for Disease Control and Prevention. *The state of aging and health in America 2013. 2013*; Available from: http://www.cdc.gov/features/agingandhealth/state_of_aging_and_health_in_america_2013.pdf.

[43] Szulc P, Kaufman JM and Orwoll ES. Osteoporosis in men. *J Osteoporos* 2012;2012:675984.

[44] Leslie WD, O'Donnell S, Jean S, Lagace C, Walsh P, Bancej C, Morin S, Hanley DA and Papaioannou A. Trends in hip fracture rates in Canada. *JAMA* 2009;302:883-9.

[45] Abrahamsen B and Vestergaard P. Declining incidence of hip fractures and the extent of use of anti-osteoporotic therapy in Denmark 1997-2006. *Osteoporos Int* 2010;21:373-80.

[46] Fisher AA, O'Brien ED and Davis MW. Trends in hip fracture epidemiology in Australia: possible impact of bisphosphonates and hormone replacement therapy. *Bone* 2009;45:246-53.

[47] Cooper C, Cole ZA, Holroyd CR, Earl SC, Harvey NC, Dennison EM, Melton LJ, Cummings SR and Kanis JA. Secular trends in the incidence of hip and other osteoporotic fractures. *Osteoporos Int* 2011;22:1277-88.

[48] Maravic M, Taupin P, Landais P and Roux C. Change in hip fracture incidence over the last 6 years in France. *Osteoporos I*nt 2011;22:797-801.

[49] Chevalley T, Guilley E, Herrmann FR, Hoffmeyer P, Rapin CH and Rizzoli R. Incidence of hip fracture over a 10-year period (1991-2000): reversal of a secular trend. *Bone* 2007;40:1284-9.

[50] Icks A, Haastert B, Wildner M, Becker C and Meyer G. Trend of hip fracture incidence in Germany 1995-2004: a population-based study. *Osteoporos Int* 2008;19:1139-45.

[51] Hagino H, Furukawa K, Fujiwara S, Okano T, Katagiri H, Yamamoto K and Teshima R. Recent trends in the incidence and lifetime risk of hip fracture in Tottori, Japan. *Osteoporos Int* 2009;20:543-8.

[52] Arias E. United States life tables, 2004. *Natl Vital Stat Rep* 2007;56:1-39.

[53] von Friesendorff M, McGuigan FE, Besjakov J and Akesson K. Hip fracture in men-survival and subsequent fractures: a cohort study with 22-year follow-up. *J Am Geriatr Soc* 2011;59:806-13.

[54] Lawrence VA, Hilsenbeck SG, Noveck H, Poses RM and Carson JL. Medical complications and outcomes after hip fracture repair. *Arch Intern Med* 2002;162:2053-7.

[55] Leslie WD and Morin SN. Osteoporosis epidemiology 2013: implications for diagnosis, risk assessment, and treatment. *Curr Opin Rheumatol* 2014;26:440-6.

[56] Ioannidis G, Flahive J, Pickard L, Papaioannou A, Chapurlat RD, Saag KG, Silverman S, Anderson FA, Jr., Gehlbach SH, Hooven FH, et al., Non-hip, non-spine fractures drive healthcare utilization following a fracture: the Global Longitudinal Study of Osteoporosis in Women (GLOW). *Osteoporos Int* 2013;24:59-67.

[57] Bliuc D, Nguyen TV, Eisman JA and Center JR. The impact of nonhip nonvertebral fractures in elderly women and men. *J Clin Endocrinol Metab* 2014;99:415-23.

[58] Exploring the biological contributions to human health: does sex matter? *J Womens Health Gend Based Med* 2001;10:433-9.

[59] Dy CJ, Lamont LE, Ton QV and Lane JM. Sex and gender considerations in male patients with osteoporosis. *Clin Orthop Relat Res* 2011;469:1906-12.

[60] Center JR, Nguyen TV, Schneider D, Sambrook PN and Eisman JA. Mortality after all major types of osteoporotic fracture in men and women: an observational study. *Lancet* 1999;353:878-82.

[61] Johnell O, Kanis J and Gullberg G. Mortality, morbidity, and assessment of fracture risk in male osteoporosis. *Calcif Tissue Int* 2001;69:182-4.

[62] Feldstein AC, Nichols G, Orwoll E, Elmer PJ, Smith DH, Herson M and Aickin M. The near absence of osteoporosis treatment in older men with fractures. *Osteoporos Int* 2005;16:953-62.

[63] Morris CA, Cabral D, Cheng H, Katz JN, Finkelstein JS, Avorn J and Solomon DH. Patterns of bone mineral density testing: current guidelines, testing rates, and interventions. *J Gen Intern Med* 2004;19:783-90.

[64] Cauley JA, Thompson DE, Ensrud KC, Scott JC and Black D. Risk of mortality following clinical fractures. *Osteoporos Int* 2000;11:556-61.

[65] Jacobsen SJ, Cooper C, Gottlieb MS, Goldberg J, Yahnke DP and Melton LJ, 3rd. Hospitalization with vertebral fracture among the aged: a national population-based study, 1986-1989. *Epidemiology* 1992;3:515-8.

[66] Furstenberg AL and Mezey MD. Differences in outcome between black and white elderly hip fracture patients. *J Chronic Dis* 1987;40:931-8.

[67] Cauley JA. Defining ethnic and racial differences in osteoporosis and fragility fractures. *Clin Orthop Relat Res* 2011;469:1891-9.

[68] Nam HS, Shin MH, Zmuda JM, Leung PC, Barrett-Connor E, Orwoll ES and Cauley JA. Race/ethnic differences in bone mineral densities in older men. *Osteoporos Int* 2010;21:2115-23.

[69] Shin MH, Zmuda JM, Barrett-Connor E, Sheu Y, Patrick AL, Leung PC, Kwok A, Kweon SS, Nam HS and Cauley JA. Race/ethnic differences in associations between bone mineral density and fracture history in older men. *Osteoporos Int* 2014;25:837-45.

[70] Karasik D, Myers RH, Cupples LA, Hannan MT, Gagnon DR, Herbert A and Kiel DP. Genome screen for quantitative trait loci

contributing to normal variation in bone mineral density: the Framingham Study. *J Bone Miner Res* 2002;17:1718-27.

[71] Van Pottelbergh I, Goemaere S, Zmierczak H, De Bacquer D and Kaufman JM. Deficient acquisition of bone during maturation underlies idiopathic osteoporosis in men: evidence from a three-generation family study. *J Bone Miner Res* 2003;18:303-11.

[72] Gennari L and Brandi ML. Genetics of male osteoporosis. *Calcif Tissue Int* 2001;69:200-4.

[73] Mackey DC, Lui LY, Cawthon PM, Bauer DC, Nevitt MC, Cauley JA, Hillier TA, Lewis CE, Barrett-Connor E and Cummings SR. High-trauma fractures and low bone mineral density in older women and men. *JAMA* 2007;298:2381-8.

[74] Amin S, Melton LJ, 3rd, Achenbach SJ, Atkinson EJ, Dekutoski MB, Kirmani S, Fischer PR and Khosla S. A distal forearm fracture in childhood is associated with an increased risk for future fragility fractures in adult men, but not women. *J Bone Miner Res* 2013;28:1751-9.

[75] Cohen-Solal ME, Baudoin C, Omouri M, Kuntz D and De Vernejoul MC. Bone mass in middle-aged osteoporotic men and their relatives: familial effect. *J Bone Miner Res* 1998;13:1909-14.

[76] Nelson RE, Nebeker JR, Sauer BC and LaFleur J. Factors associated with screening or treatment initiation among male United States veterans at risk for osteoporosis fracture. *Bone* 2012;50:983-8.

[77] Denosumab (Prolia): Treatment to Increase Bone Mass in Men with Osteoporosis at High Risk for Fracture; or Who Have Failed or are Intolerant to Other Available Osteoporosis Therapy: Ottawa (ON) *Common Drug Review.* Canadian Agency for Drugs and Technologies in Health; 2015 Oct.

[78] Szulc P, Blackwell T, Kiel DP, Schousboe JT, Cauley J, Hillier T, Hochberg M, Rodondi N, Taylor BC, Black D, et al., Abdominal aortic calcification and risk of fracture among older women - The SOF study. *Bone* 2015;81:16-23.

[79] Cauley JA, Cawthon PM, Peters KE, Cummings SR, Ensrud KE, Bauer DC, Taylor BC, Shikany JM, Hoffman AR, Lane NE, et al.,

Risk Factors for Hip Fracture in Older Men: The Osteoporotic Fractures in Men Study (MrOS). *J Bone Miner Res* 2016;31:1810-1819.

[80] Ensrud KE, Taylor BC, Paudel ML, Cauley JA, Cawthon PM, Cummings SR, Fink HA, Barrett-Connor E, Zmuda JM, Shikany JM, et al., Serum 25-hydroxyvitamin D levels and rate of hip bone loss in older men. *J Clin Endocrinol Metab* 2009;94:2773-80.

[81] Cauley JA, Parimi N, Ensrud KE, Bauer DC, Cawthon PM, Cummings SR, Hoffman AR, Shikany JM, Barrett-Connor E and Orwoll E. Serum 25-hydroxyvitamin D and the risk of hip and nonspine fractures in older men. *J Bone Miner Res* 2010;25:545-53.

[82] Cauley JA, Ewing SK, Taylor BC, Fink HA, Ensrud KE, Bauer DC, Barrett-Connor E, Marshall L and Orwoll ES. Sex steroid hormones in older men: longitudinal associations with 4.5-year change in hip bone mineral density--the osteoporotic fractures in men study. *J Clin Endocrinol Metab* 2010;95:4314-23.

[83] LeBlanc ES, Nielson CM, Marshall LM, Lapidus JA, Barrett-Connor E, Ensrud KE, Hoffman AR, Laughlin G, Ohlsson C and Orwoll ES. The effects of serum testosterone, estradiol, and sex hormone binding globulin levels on fracture risk in older men. *J Clin Endocrinol Metab* 2009;94:3337-46.

[84] Barrett-Connor E, Laughlin GA, Li H, Nielson CM, Wang PY, Dam TT, Cauley JA, Ensrud KE, Stefanick ML, Lau E, et al., The association of concurrent vitamin D and sex hormone deficiency with bone loss and fracture risk in older men: the osteoporotic fractures in men (MrOS) study. *J Bone Miner Res* 2012;27:2306-13.

[85] Curtis JR, Ewing SK, Bauer DC, Cauley JA, Cawthon PM, Barrett-Connor E, Haney EM, Ishani A, Cremers S and Orwoll E. Association of intact parathyroid hormone levels with subsequent hip BMD loss: the Osteoporotic Fractures in Men (MrOS) Study. *J Clin Endocrinol Metab* 2012;97:1937-44.

[86] Diem SJ, Harrison SL, Haney E, Cauley JA, Stone KL, Orwoll E and Ensrud KE. Depressive symptoms and rates of bone loss at the hip in older men. *Osteoporos Int* 2013;24:111-9.

[87] Fink HA, Harrison SL, Taylor BC, Cummings SR, Schousboe JT, Kuskowski MA, Stone KL and Ensrud KE. Differences in site-specific fracture risk among older women with discordant results for osteoporosis at hip and spine: study of osteoporotic fractures. *J Clin Densitom* 2008;11:250-9.

[88] Williams FM, Cherkas LF, Spector TD and MacGregor AJ. The effect of moderate alcohol consumption on bone mineral density: a study of female twins. *Ann Rheum Dis* 2005;64:309-10.

[89] Berg KM, Kunins HV, Jackson JL, Nahvi S, Chaudhry A, Harris KA, Jr., Malik R and Arnsten JH. Association between alcohol consumption and both osteoporotic fracture and bone density. *Am J Med* 2008;121:406-18.

[90] Hoidrup S, Gronbaek M, Gottschau A, Lauritzen JB and Schroll M. Alcohol intake, beverage preference, and risk of hip fracture in men and women. Copenhagen Centre for Prospective Population Studies. *Am J Epidemiol* 1999;149:993-1001.

[91] Fanti P, Monier-Faugere MC, Geng Z, Cohen D and Malluche HH. Moderately high consumption of ethanol suppresses bone resorption in ovariectomized but not in sexually intact adult female rats. *Alcohol Clin Exp Res* 1997;21:1150-4.

[92] Poli A, Marangoni F, Avogaro A, Barba G, Bellentani S, Bucci M, Cambieri R, Catapano AL, Costanzo S, Cricelli C, et al., Moderate alcohol use and health: a consensus document. *Nutr Metab Cardiovasc Dis* 2013;23:487-504.

[93] Flegal KM, Carroll MD, Ogden CL and Curtin LR. Prevalence and trends in obesity among US adults, 1999-2008. *JAMA* 2010;303:235-41.

[94] Sundquist J, Johansson SE and Sundquist K. Levelling off of prevalence of obesity in the adult population of Sweden between 2000/01 and 2004/05. *BMC Public Health* 2010;10:119.

[95] Haby MM, Markwick A, Peeters A, Shaw J and Vos T. Future predictions of body mass index and overweight prevalence in Australia, 2005-2025. *Health Promot Int* 2012;27:250-60.

[96] Finucane MM, Stevens GA, Cowan MJ, Danaei G, Lin JK, Paciorek CJ, Singh GM, Gutierrez HR, Lu Y, Bahalim AN, et al., National, regional, and global trends in body-mass index since 1980: systematic analysis of health examination surveys and epidemiological studies with 960 country-years and 9.1 million participants. *Lancet* 2011;377:557-67.

[97] Sogaard AJ, Holvik K, Omsland TK, Tell GS, Dahl C, Schei B, Falch JA, Eisman JA and Meyer HE. Abdominal obesity increases the risk of hip fracture. A population-based study of 43,000 women and men aged 60-79 years followed for 8 years. Cohort of Norway. *J Intern Med* 2015;277:306-17.

[98] Bredella MA, Lin E, Gerweck AV, Landa MG, Thomas BJ, Torriani M, Bouxsein ML and Miller KK. Determinants of bone microarchitecture and mechanical properties in obese men. *J Clin Endocrinol Metab* 2012;97:4115-22.

[99] Scott D, Seibel M, Cumming R, Naganathan V, Blyth F, Le Couteur DG, Handelsman DJ, Waite LM and Hirani V. Sarcopenic Obesity and Its Temporal Associations With Changes in Bone Mineral Density, Incident Falls, and Fractures in Older Men: The Concord Health and Ageing in Men Project. *J Bone Miner Res* 2017;32:575-583.

[100] Napoli N, Strotmeyer ES, Ensrud KE, Sellmeyer DE, Bauer DC, Hoffman AR, Dam TT, Barrett-Connor E, Palermo L, Orwoll ES, et al., Fracture risk in diabetic elderly men: the MrOS study. *Diabetologia* 2014;57:2057-65.

[101] Cohen A, Dempster DW, Recker RR, Lappe JM, Zhou H, Zwahlen A, Muller R, Zhao B, Guo X, Lang T, et al., Abdominal fat is associated with lower bone formation and inferior bone quality in healthy premenopausal women: a transiliac bone biopsy study. *J Clin Endocrinol Metab* 2013;98:2562-72.

[102] Arikan S, Tuzcu A, Bahceci M, Ozmen S and Gokalp D. Insulin resistance in type 2 diabetes mellitus may be related to bone mineral density. *J Clin Densitom* 2012;15:186-90.

[103] Terzi R, Dindar S, Terzi H and Demirtas O. Relationships among the metabolic syndrome, bone mineral density, bone turnover markers, and hyperglycemia. *Metab Syndr Relat Disord* 2015;13:78-83.
[104] Mandal CC. High Cholesterol Deteriorates Bone Health: New Insights into Molecular Mechanisms. *Front Endocrinol* (Lausanne) 2015;6:165.
[105] Yamauchi M, Yamaguchi T, Nawata K, Tanaka K, Takaoka S and Sugimoto T. Increased low-density lipoprotein cholesterol level is associated with non-vertebral fractures in postmenopausal women. *Endocrine* 2015;48:279-86.
[106] Ramos-Junior ES, Leite GA, Carmo-Silva CC, Taira TM, Neves KB, Colon DF, da Silva LA, Salvador SL, Tostes RC, Cunha FQ, et al., Adipokine Chemerin Bridges Metabolic Dyslipidemia and Alveolar Bone Loss in Mice. *J Bone Miner Res* 2016.
[107] Pelton K, Krieder J, Joiner D, Freeman MR, Goldstein SA and Solomon KR. Hypercholesterolemia promotes an osteoporotic phenotype. *Am J Pathol* 2012;181:928-36.
[108] You L, Sheng ZY, Tang CL, Chen L, Pan L and Chen JY. High cholesterol diet increases osteoporosis risk via inhibiting bone formation in rats. *Acta Pharmacol Sin* 2011;32:1498-504.
[109] Chen JR, Zhang J, Lazarenko OP, Cao JJ, Blackburn ML, Badger TM and Ronis MJ. Soy protein isolates prevent loss of bone quantity associated with obesity in rats through regulation of insulin signaling in osteoblasts. *FASEB J* 2013;27:3514-23.
[110] Yamamoto T, Ozono K, Miyauchi A, Kasayama S, Kojima Y, Shima M and Okada S. Role of advanced glycation end products in adynamic bone disease in patients with diabetic nephropathy. *Am J Kidney Dis* 2001;38:S161-4.
[111] Odetti P, Rossi S, Monacelli F, Poggi A, Cirnigliaro M, Federici M and Federici A. Advanced glycation end products and bone loss during aging. *Ann N Y Acad Sci* 2005;1043:710-7.
[112] Drake MT, Murad MH, Mauck KF, Lane MA, Undavalli C, Elraiyah T, Stuart LM, Prasad C, Shahrour A, Mullan RJ, et al., Clinical review. Risk factors for low bone mass-related fractures in men: a

systematic review and meta-analysis. *J Clin Endocrinol Metab* 2012;97:1861-70.

[113] Olofsson H, Byberg L, Mohsen R, Melhus H, Lithell H and Michaelsson K. Smoking and the risk of fracture in older men. *J Bone Miner Res* 2005;20:1208-15.

[114] Pompe E, Bartstra J, Verhaar HJ, de Koning HJ, van der Aalst CM, Oudkerk M, Vliegenthart R, Lammers JJ, de Jong PA and Mohamed Hoesein FA. Bone density loss on computed tomography at 3-year follow-up in current compared to former male smokers. *Eur J Radiol* 2017;89:177-181.

[115] Felson DT, Kiel DP, Anderson JJ and Kannel WB. Alcohol consumption and hip fractures: the Framingham Study. *Am J Epidemiol* 1988;128:1102-10.

[116] Jepsen KJ. Systems analysis of bone. *Wiley Interdiscip Rev Syst Biol Med* 2009;1:73-88.

[117] Lespessailles E, Cortet B, Legrand E, Guggenbuhl P and Roux C. Low-trauma fractures without osteoporosis. *Osteoporos Int* 2017.

[118] Riggs BL, Melton Iii LJ, 3rd, Robb RA, Camp JJ, Atkinson EJ, Peterson JM, Rouleau PA, McCollough CH, Bouxsein ML and Khosla S. Population-based study of age and sex differences in bone volumetric density, size, geometry, and structure at different skeletal sites. *J Bone Miner Res* 2004;19:1945-54.

[119] Riggs BL. Endocrine causes of age-related bone loss and osteoporosis. *Novartis Found Symp* 2002;242:247-59*; discussion* 260-4.

[120] Silva MJ and Gibson LJ. Modeling the mechanical behavior of vertebral trabecular bone: effects of age-related changes in microstructure. *Bone* 1997;21:191-9.

[121] Zebaze RM, Ghasem-Zadeh A, Bohte A, Iuliano-Burns S, Mirams M, Price RI, Mackie EJ and Seeman E. Intracortical remodelling and porosity in the distal radius and post-mortem femurs of women: a cross-sectional study. *Lancet* 2010;375:1729-36.

[122] Almeida M, Laurent MR, Dubois V, Claessens F, O'Brien CA, Bouillon R, Vanderschueren D and Manolagas SC. Estrogens and

Androgens in Skeletal Physiology and Pathophysiology. *Physiol Rev* 2017;97:135-187.

[123] Manolagas SC. Birth and death of bone cells: basic regulatory mechanisms and implications for the pathogenesis and treatment of osteoporosis. *Endocr Rev* 2000;21:115-37.

[124] Manolagas SC, Kousteni S and Jilka RL. Sex steroids and bone. *Recent Prog Horm Res* 2002;57:385-409.

[125] Gennari L and Bilezikian JP. Idiopathic osteoporosis in men. *Curr Osteoporos Rep* 2013;11:286-98.

[126] Gennari L and Bilezikian JP. Osteoporosis in men: pathophysiology and treatment. *Curr Rheumatol Rep* 2007;9:71-7.

[127] Khosla S, Melton LJ, 3rd, Achenbach SJ, Oberg AL and Riggs BL. Hormonal and biochemical determinants of trabecular microstructure at the ultradistal radius in women and men. *J Clin Endocrinol Metab* 2006;91:885-91.

[128] Khosla S. Estrogen and bone: insights from estrogen-resistant, aromatase-deficient, and normal men. *Bone* 2008;43:414-7.

[129] Harman SM, Metter EJ, Tobin JD, Pearson J and Blackman MR. Longitudinal effects of aging on serum total and free testosterone levels in healthy men. Baltimore Longitudinal Study of Aging. *J Clin Endocrinol Metab* 2001;86:724-31.

[130] Kousteni S, Chen JR, Bellido T, Han L, Ali AA, O'Brien CA, Plotkin L, Fu Q, Mancino AT, Wen Y, et al., Reversal of bone loss in mice by nongenotropic signaling of sex steroids. *Science* 2002;298:843-6.

[131] Tomkinson A, Reeve J, Shaw RW and Noble BS. The death of osteocytes via apoptosis accompanies estrogen withdrawal in human bone. *J Clin Endocrinol Metab* 1997;82:3128-35.

[132] Tomkinson A, Gevers EF, Wit JM, Reeve J and Noble BS. The role of estrogen in the control of rat osteocyte apoptosis. *J Bone Miner Res* 1998;13:1243-50.

[133] Fink HA, Ewing SK, Ensrud KE, Barrett-Connor E, Taylor BC, Cauley JA and Orwoll ES. Association of testosterone and estradiol deficiency with osteoporosis and rapid bone loss in older men. *J Clin Endocrinol Metab* 2006;91:3908-15.

[134] Khosla S, Melton LJ, 3rd and Riggs BL. Clinical review 144: Estrogen and the male skeleton. *J Clin Endocrinol Metab* 2002;87:1443-50.

[135] Gennari L, Nuti R and Bilezikian JP. Aromatase activity and bone homeostasis in men. *J Clin Endocrinol Metab* 2004;89:5898-907.

[136] Gennari L, Khosla S and Bilezikian JP. Estrogen and fracture risk in men. *J Bone Miner Res* 2008;23:1548-51.

[137] Wiren KM, Zhang XW, Olson DA, Turner RT and Iwaniec UT. Androgen prevents hypogonadal bone loss via inhibition of resorption mediated by mature osteoblasts/osteocytes. *Bone* 2012;51:835-46.

[138] Guntur AR and Rosen CJ. IGF-1 regulation of key signaling pathways in bone. *Bonekey Rep* 2013;2:437.

[139] Crane JL and Cao X. Function of matrix IGF-1 in coupling bone resorption and formation. *J Mol Med* (Berl) 2014;92:107-15.

[140] Xian L, Wu X, Pang L, Lou M, Rosen CJ, Qiu T, Crane J, Frassica F, Zhang L, Rodriguez JP, et al., Matrix IGF-1 maintains bone mass by activation of mTOR in mesenchymal stem cells. *Nat Med* 2012;18:1095-101.

[141] Nicolas V, Prewett A, Bettica P, Mohan S, Finkelman RD, Baylink DJ and Farley JR. Age-related decreases in insulin-like growth factor-I and transforming growth factor-beta in femoral cortical bone from both men and women: implications for bone loss with aging. *J Clin Endocrinol Metab* 1994;78:1011-6.

[142] Seck T, Scheppach B, Scharla S, Diel I, Blum WF, Bismar H, Schmid G, Krempien B, Ziegler R and Pfeilschifter J. Concentration of insulin-like growth factor (IGF)-I and -II in iliac crest bone matrix from pre- and postmenopausal women: relationship to age, menopause, bone turnover, bone volume, and circulating IGFs. *J Clin Endocrinol Metab* 1998;83:2331-7.

[143] Ohlsson C, Mellstrom D, Carlzon D, Orwoll E, Ljunggren O, Karlsson MK and Vandenput L. Older men with low serum IGF-1 have an increased risk of incident fractures: the MrOS Sweden study. *J Bone Miner Res* 2011;26:865-72.

[144] Dashkova I, Dashkova A, Kozikowski A, Gupta A, Sison C, Ibrahim R, Sinvani L, Pekmezaris R and Wolf-Klein G. Differences According to Sex in Perspectives and Beliefs on Osteoporosis: A Cross-Sectional Survey Study. *J Am Geriatr Soc* 2016;64:e85-e86.

[145] Cummings SR, Cawthon PM, Ensrud KE, Cauley JA, Fink HA and Orwoll ES. BMD and risk of hip and nonvertebral fractures in older men: a prospective study and comparison with older women. *J Bone Miner Res* 2006;21:1550-6.

[146] Szulc P, Munoz F, Duboeuf F, Marchand F and Delmas PD. Bone mineral density predicts osteoporotic fractures in elderly men: the MINOS study. *Osteoporos Int* 2005;16:1184-92.

[147] O'Connor KM. Evaluation and Treatment of Osteoporosis. *Med Clin North Am* 2016;100:807-26.

[148] Kanis JA, Oden A, Johansson H, Borgstrom F, Strom O and McCloskey E. FRAX and its applications to clinical practice. *Bone* 2009;44:734-43.

[149] Nguyen ND, Frost SA, Center JR, Eisman JA and Nguyen TV. Development of a nomogram for individualizing hip fracture risk in men and women. *Osteoporos Int* 2007;18:1109-17.

[150] Blaizot S, Delmas PD, Marchand F, Chapurlat R and Szulc P. Risk factors for peripheral fractures vary by age in older men--the prospective MINOS study. *Osteoporos Int* 2011;22:1755-64.

[151] Sandhu SK, Nguyen ND, Center JR, Pocock NA, Eisman JA and Nguyen TV. Prognosis of fracture: evaluation of predictive accuracy of the FRAX algorithm and Garvan nomogram. *Osteoporos Int* 2010;21:863-71.

[152] Silva DR, Coelho AC, Dumke A, Valentini JD, de Nunes JN, Stefani CL, da Silva Mendes LF and Knorst MM. Osteoporosis prevalence and associated factors in patients with COPD: a cross-sectional study. *Respir Care* 2011;56:961-8.

[153] Morden NE, Sullivan SD, Bartle B and Lee TA. Skeletal health in men with chronic lung disease: rates of testing, treatment, and fractures. *Osteoporos Int* 2011;22:1855-62.

[154] Shen C, Deng J, Zhou R, Chen J, Fan S, Li Z, Hu Y and Zhong Q. Relation between bone mineral density, bone loss and the risk of cardiovascular disease in a Chinese cohort. *Am J Cardiol* 2012;110:1138-42.
[155] Roux C. Osteoporosis in inflammatory joint diseases. *Osteoporos Int* 2011;22:421-33.
[156] Castano-Betancourt MC, Rivadeneira F, Bierma-Zeinstra S, Kerkhof HJ, Hofman A, Uitterlinden AG and van Meurs JB. Bone parameters across different types of hip osteoarthritis and their relationship to osteoporotic fracture risk. *Arthritis Rheum* 2013;65:693-700.
[157] Hearn AP and Silber E. Osteoporosis in multiple sclerosis. *Mult Scler* 2010;16:1031-43.
[158] Krela-Kazmierczak I, Szymczak A, Lykowska-Szuber L, Eder P and Linke K. Osteoporosis in Gastrointestinal Diseases. *Adv Clin Exp Med* 2016;25:185-90.
[159] Sidlauskas KM, Sutton EE and Biddle MA. Osteoporosis in men: epidemiology and treatment with denosumab. *Clin Interv Aging* 2014;9:593-601.
[160] Feldstein A, Elmer PJ, Smith DH, Herson M, Orwoll E, Chen C, Aickin M and Swain MC. Electronic medical record reminder improves osteoporosis management after a fracture: a randomized, controlled trial. *J Am Geriatr Soc* 2006;54:450-7.
[161] Adler RA. Management of osteoporosis in men on androgen deprivation therapy. *Maturitas* 2011;68:143-7.
[162] Black DM and Rosen CJ. Clinical Practice. Postmenopausal Osteoporosis. *N Engl J Med* 2016;374:254-62.
[163] Haentjens P, Johnell O, Kanis JA, Bouillon R, Cooper C, Lamraski G, Vanderschueren D, Kaufman JM and Boonen S. Evidence from data searches and life-table analyses for gender-related differences in absolute risk of hip fracture after Colles' or spine fracture: Colles' fracture as an early and sensitive marker of skeletal fragility in white men. *J Bone Miner Res* 2004;19:1933-44.

[164] Chitre MM and Hayes W. 3-year results of a member and physician intervention to reduce risk associated with glucocorticoid-induced osteoporosis in a health plan. *J Manag Care Pharm* 2008;14:281-90.

[165] Brown JE, Sherriff JM and James ND. Osteoporosis in patients with prostate cancer on long-term androgen deprivation therapy: an increasing, but under-recognized problem. *BJU Int* 2010;105:1042-3.

[166] National Osteoporosis Foundation. *Clinician's Guide to Prevention and Treatment of Osteoporosis*. 2014 [cited 2017; Available from: http://nof.org/hcp/clinicians-guide.

[167] Watts NB, Adler RA, Bilezikian JP, Drake MT, Eastell R, Orwoll ES and Finkelstein JS. Osteoporosis in men: an Endocrine Society clinical practice guideline. *J Clin Endocrinol Metab* 2012;97:1802-22.

[168] Black DM and Rosen CJ. Postmenopausal Osteoporosis. *N Engl J Med* 2016;374:2096-7.

[169] Bauer DC. Clinical practice. Calcium supplements and fracture prevention. *N Engl J Med* 2013;369:1537-43.

[170] Murad MH, Drake MT, Mullan RJ, Mauck KF, Stuart LM, Lane MA, Abu Elnour NO, Erwin PJ, Hazem A, Puhan MA, et al., Clinical review. Comparative effectiveness of drug treatments to prevent fragility fractures: a systematic review and network meta-analysis. *J Clin Endocrinol Metab* 2012;97:1871-80.

[171] LeBlanc ES and Chou R. Vitamin D and falls-fitting new data with current guidelines. *JAMA Intern Med* 2015;175:712-3.

[172] Sanders KM, Stuart AL, Williamson EJ, Simpson JA, Kotowicz MA, Young D and Nicholson GC. Annual high-dose oral vitamin D and falls and fractures in older women: a randomized controlled trial. *JAMA* 2010;303:1815-22.

[173] Smith H, Anderson F, Raphael H, Maslin P, Crozier S and Cooper C. Effect of annual intramuscular vitamin D on fracture risk in elderly men and women--a population-based, randomized, double-blind, placebo-controlled trial. *Rheumatology* (Oxford) 2007;46:1852-7.

[174] Bischoff-Ferrari HA, Dawson-Hughes B, Orav EJ, Staehelin HB, Meyer OW, Theiler R, Dick W, Willett WC and Egli A. Monthly

High-Dose Vitamin D Treatment for the Prevention of Functional Decline: A Randomized Clinical Trial. *JAMA Intern Med* 2016; 176:175-83.

[175] Gallagher JC. Letter to the editor. *Menopause* 2015;22:579.

[176] Institute of Medicine, *Dietary Reference Intakes for Calcium and Vitamin D*, A.C. Ross, Taylor, C.L., Yaktine, A.L., Del Valle, H.B., Editor 2011, Institute of Medicine: Washington, DC.

[177] Tosi LL, Boyan BD and Boskey AL. Does sex matter in musculoskeletal health? The influence of sex and gender on musculoskeletal health. *J Bone Joint Surg Am* 2005;87:1631-47.

[178] O'Connor KM and Paauw DS. Pharmacologic Therapies: Updates and Clinical Pearls. *Med Clin North Am* 2016;100:xvii-xviii.

[179] Crandall CJ, Newberry SJ, Diamant A, Lim YW, Gellad WF, Booth MJ, Motala A and Shekelle PG. Comparative effectiveness of pharmacologic treatments to prevent fractures: an updated systematic review. *Ann Intern Med* 2014;161:711-23.

[180] Khosla S, Bilezikian JP, Dempster DW, Lewiecki EM, Miller PD, Neer RM, Recker RR, Shane E, Shoback D and Potts JT. Benefits and risks of bisphosphonate therapy for osteoporosis. *J Clin Endocrinol Metab* 2012;97:2272-82.

[181] Boonen S, Reginster JY, Kaufman JM, Lippuner K, Zanchetta J, Langdahl B, Rizzoli R, Lipschitz S, Dimai HP, Witvrouw R, et al., Fracture risk and zoledronic acid therapy in men with osteoporosis. *N Engl J Med* 2012;367:1714-23.

[182] Lyles KW, Colon-Emeric CS, Magaziner JS, Adachi JD, Pieper CF, Mautalen C, Hyldstrup L, Recknor C, Nordsletten L, Moore KA, et al., Zoledronic acid and clinical fractures and mortality after hip fracture. *N Engl J Med* 2007;357:1799-809.

[183] Shane E, Burr D, Abrahamsen B, Adler RA, Brown TD, Cheung AM, Cosman F, Curtis JR, Dell R, Dempster DW, et al., Atypical subtrochanteric and diaphyseal femoral fractures: second report of a task force of the American Society for Bone and Mineral Research. *J Bone Miner Res* 2014;29:1-23.

[184] Khan AA, Morrison A, Hanley DA, Felsenberg D, McCauley LK, O'Ryan F, Reid IR, Ruggiero SL, Taguchi A, Tetradis S, et al., Diagnosis and management of osteonecrosis of the jaw: a systematic review and international consensus. *J Bone Miner Res* 2015;30:3-23.

[185] Orwoll E, Teglbjaerg CS, Langdahl BL, Chapurlat R, Czerwinski E, Kendler DL, Reginster JY, Kivitz A, Lewiecki EM, Miller PD, et al., A randomized, placebo-controlled study of the effects of denosumab for the treatment of men with low bone mineral density. *J Clin Endocrinol Metab* 2012;97:3161-9.

[186] In Denosumab versus Zoledronic Acid for Adults with Osteoporosis: *A Review of Cost-Effectiveness* 2016: Ottawa (ON).

[187] Cawthon PM, Shahnazari M, Orwoll ES and Lane NE. Osteoporosis in men: findings from the Osteoporotic Fractures in Men Study (MrOS). *Ther Adv Musculoskelet Dis* 2016;8:15-27.

[188] Smith MR, Egerdie B, Hernandez Toriz N, Feldman R, Tammela TL, Saad F, Heracek J, Szwedowski M, Ke C, Kupic A, et al., Denosumab in men receiving androgen-deprivation therapy for prostate cancer. *N Engl J Med* 2009;361:745-55.

[189] Cusano NE, Costa AG, Silva BC and Bilezikian JP. Therapy of osteoporosis in men with teriparatide. *J Osteoporos* 2011;2011:463675.

[190] Neer RM, Arnaud CD, Zanchetta JR, Prince R, Gaich GA, Reginster JY, Hodsman AB, Eriksen EF, Ish-Shalom S, Genant HK, et al., Effect of parathyroid hormone (1-34) on fractures and bone mineral density in postmenopausal women with osteoporosis. *N Engl J Med* 2001;344:1434-41.

[191] Orwoll ES, Scheele WH, Paul S, Adami S, Syversen U, Diez-Perez A, Kaufman JM, Clancy AD and Gaich GA. The effect of teriparatide [human parathyroid hormone (1-34)] therapy on bone density in men with osteoporosis. *J Bone Miner Res* 2003;18:9-17.

[192] Saag KG, Zanchetta JR, Devogelaer JP, Adler RA, Eastell R, See K, Krege JH, Krohn K and Warner MR. Effects of teriparatide versus alendronate for treating glucocorticoid-induced osteoporosis: thirty-

six-month results of a randomized, double-blind, controlled trial. *Arthritis Rheum* 2009;60:3346-55.

[193] Gedmintas L, Solomon DH and Kim SC. Bisphosphonates and risk of subtrochanteric, femoral shaft, and atypical femur fracture: a systematic review and meta-analysis. *J Bone Miner Res* 2013;28: 1729-37.

[194] Adler RA. Duration of anti-resorptive therapy for osteoporosis. *Endocrine* 2016;51:222-4.

[195] Black DM, Schwartz AV, Ensrud KE, Cauley JA, Levis S, Quandt SA, Satterfield S, Wallace RB, Bauer DC, Palermo L, et al., Effects of continuing or stopping alendronate after 5 years of treatment: the Fracture Intervention Trial Long-term Extension (FLEX): a randomized trial. *JAMA* 2006;296:2927-38.

[196] Black DM, Reid IR, Boonen S, Bucci-Rechtweg C, Cauley JA, Cosman F, Cummings SR, Hue TF, Lippuner K, Lakatos P, et al., The effect of 3 versus 6 years of zoledronic acid treatment of osteoporosis: a randomized extension to the HORIZON-Pivotal Fracture Trial (PFT). *J Bone Miner Res* 2012;27:243-54.

[197] Black DM, Bauer DC, Schwartz AV, Cummings SR and Rosen CJ. Continuing bisphosphonate treatment for osteoporosis--for whom and for how long? *N Engl J Med* 2012;366:2051-3.

[198] Cosman F, Cauley JA, Eastell R, Boonen S, Palermo L, Reid IR, Cummings SR and Black DM. Reassessment of fracture risk in women after 3 years of treatment with zoledronic acid: when is it reasonable to discontinue treatment? *J Clin Endocrinol Metab* 2014;99:4546-54.

[199] Reid IR. Controversies in osteoporosis management. *Intern Med J* 2016;46:767-70.

[200] Chesnut CH, 3rd, Skag A, Christiansen C, Recker R, Stakkestad JA, Hoiseth A, Felsenberg D, Huss H, Gilbride J, Schimmer RC, et al., Effects of oral ibandronate administered daily or intermittently on fracture risk in postmenopausal osteoporosis. *J Bone Miner Res* 2004;19:1241-9.

[201] Cummings SR, San Martin J, McClung MR, Siris ES, Eastell R, Reid IR, Delmas P, Zoog HB, Austin M, Wang A, et al., Denosumab for prevention of fractures in postmenopausal women with osteoporosis. *N Engl J Med* 2009;361:756-65.

[202] Greenspan SL, Bone HG, Ettinger MP, Hanley DA, Lindsay R, Zanchetta JR, Blosch CM, Mathisen AL, Morris SA and Marriott TB. Effect of recombinant human parathyroid hormone (1-84) on vertebral fracture and bone mineral density in postmenopausal women with osteoporosis: a randomized trial. *Ann Intern Med* 2007;146:326-39.

[203] Eiken P and Vestergaard P. Treatment of osteoporosis after alendronate or risedronate. *Osteoporos Int* 2016;27:1-12.

[204] Roux C, Hofbauer LC, Ho PR, Wark JD, Zillikens MC, Fahrleitner-Pammer A, Hawkins F, Micaelo M, Minisola S, Papaioannou N, et al., Denosumab compared with risedronate in postmenopausal women suboptimally adherent to alendronate therapy: efficacy and safety results from a randomized open-label study. *Bone* 2014;58:48-54.

[205] Freemantle N, Satram-Hoang S, Tang ET, Kaur P, Macarios D, Siddhanti S, Borenstein J and Kendler DL. Final results of the DAPS (Denosumab Adherence Preference Satisfaction) study: a 24-month, randomized, crossover comparison with alendronate in postmenopausal women. *Osteoporos Int* 2012;23:317-26.

[206] Cosman F, Dempster DW, Nieves JW, Zhou H, Zion M, Roimisher C, Houle Y, Lindsay R and Bostrom M. Effect of Teriparatide on Bone Formation in the Human Femoral Neck. *J Clin Endocrinol Metab* 2016;101:1498-505.

[207] Cosman F, Nieves JW and Dempster DW. Treatment Sequence Matters: Anabolic and Antiresorptive Therapy for Osteoporosis. *J Bone Miner Res* 2017;32:198-202.

[208] McClung MR. Emerging Therapies for Osteoporosis. *Endocrinol Metab (Seoul)* 2015;30:429-35.

[209] Kenny AM, Kleppinger A, Annis K, Rathier M, Browner B, Judge JO and McGee D. Effects of transdermal testosterone on bone and

muscle in older men with low bioavailable testosterone levels, low bone mass, and physical frailty. *J Am Geriatr Soc* 2010;58:1134-43.

[210] Snyder PJ, Kopperdahl DL, Stephens-Shields AJ, Ellenberg SS, Cauley JA, Ensrud KE, Lewis CE, Barrett-Connor E, Schwartz AV, Lee DC, et al., Effect of Testosterone Treatment on Volumetric Bone Density and Strength in Older Men With Low Testosterone: A Controlled Clinical Trial. *JAMA Intern Med* 2017.

[211] Seftel AD. Re: Testosterone Products: Drug Safety Communication - FDA Cautions about Using Testosterone Products for Low Testosterone due to Aging; Requires Labeling Change to Inform of Possible Increased Risk of Heart Attack and Stroke. *J Urol* 2015;194:759-60.

[212] Fourie H, Floyd S and Marshall B. Exploring New Zealand orthopaedic nurses' knowledge of osteoporosis. *Orthop Nurs* 2015;34:29-35.

[213] Fogelman Y, Goldshtein I, Segal E and Ish-Shalom S. Managing Osteoporosis: A Survey of Knowledge, Attitudes and Practices among Primary Care Physicians in Israel. *PLoS One* 2016; 11:e0160661.

[214] Chenot R, Scheidt-Nave C, Gabler S, Kochen MM and Himmel W. German primary care doctors' awareness of osteoporosis and knowledge of national guidelines. *Exp Clin Endocrinol Diabetes* 2007;115:584-9.

[215] Perez-Edo L, Ciria Recasens M, Castelo-Branco C, Orozco Lopez P, Gimeno Marques A, Perez C and Manasanch Dalmau J. Management of osteoporosis in general practice: a cross-sectional survey of primary care practitioners in Spain. *Osteoporos Int* 2004;15:252-7.

[216] Werner P and Vered I. Management of osteoporosis: a survey of Israeli physicians' knowledge and attitudes. *Isr Med Assoc J* 2000;2:361-4.

[217] Taylor JC, Sterkel B, Utley M, Shipley M, Newman S, Horton M and Fitz-Clarence H. Opinions and experiences in general practice on osteoporosis prevention, diagnosis and management. *Osteoporos Int* 2001;12:844-8.

[218] Bass E, French DD, Bradham DD and Rubenstein LZ. Risk-adjusted mortality rates of elderly veterans with hip fractures. *Ann Epidemiol* 2007;17:514-9.

[219] Haentjens P, Magaziner J, Colon-Emeric CS, Vanderschueren D, Milisen K, Velkeniers B and Boonen S. Meta-analysis: excess mortality after hip fracture among older women and men. *Ann Intern Med* 2010;152:380-90.

[220] Gaines JM and Marx KA. Older men's knowledge about osteoporosis and educational interventions to increase osteoporosis knowledge in older men: a systematic review. *Maturitas* 2011;68:5-12.

[221] Gaines JM, Marx KA, Narrett M, Caudill J, Landsman J and Parrish JM. Validation of the male osteoporosis knowledge quiz. *Am J Mens Health* 2011;5:78-83.

[222] Gaines JM, Marx KA, Caudill J, Parrish S, Landsman J, Narrett M and Parrish JM. Older men's knowledge of osteoporosis and the prevalence of risk factors. *J Clin Densitom* 2010;13:204-9.

[223] Bombak AE and Hanson HM. Qualitative Insights from the Osteoporosis Research: A Narrative Review of the Literature. *J Osteoporos* 2016;2016:7915041.

[224] Nielsen DS, Brixen K and Huniche L. Men's experiences of living with osteoporosis: focus group interviews. *Am J Mens Health* 2011;5:166-76.

[225] Neuman MD, Ibrahim SA, Barg FA, Osigwe C and Karlawish JH. Race and patient preferences for hip fracture care. *J Am Geriatr Soc* 2013;61:468-70.

[226] Besser SJ, Anderson JE and Weinman J. How do osteoporosis patients perceive their illness and treatment? Implications for clinical practice. *Arch Osteoporos* 2012;7:115-24.

[227] Sale JE, Bogoch E, Hawker G, Gignac M, Beaton D, Jaglal S and Frankel L. Patient perceptions of provider barriers to post-fracture secondary prevention. *Osteoporos Int* 2014;25:2581-9.

[228] Lau E, Papaioannou A, Dolovich L, Adachi J, Sawka AM, Burns S, Nair K and Pathak A. Patients' adherence to osteoporosis therapy:

exploring the perceptions of postmenopausal women. *Can Fam Physician* 2008;54:394-402.

[229] Unson CG, Siccion E, Gaztambide J, Gaztambide S, Mahoney Trella P and Prestwood K. Nonadherence and osteoporosis treatment preferences of older women: a qualitative study. *J Womens Health (Larchmt)* 2003;12:1037-45.

[230] Sahni S, Mangano KM, McLean RR, Hannan MT and Kiel DP. Dietary Approaches for Bone Health: Lessons from the Framingham Osteoporosis Study. *Curr Osteoporos Rep* 2015;13:245-55.

[231] Movassagh EZ and Vatanparast H. Current Evidence on the Association of Dietary Patterns and Bone Health: A Scoping Review. *Adv Nutr* 2017;8:1-16.

[232] Haring B, Crandall CJ, Wu C, LeBlanc ES, Shikany JM, Carbone L, Orchard T, Thomas F, Wactawaski-Wende J, Li W, et al., Dietary Patterns and Fractures in Postmenopausal Women: Results From the Women's Health Initiative. *JAMA Intern Med* 2016;176:645-52.

[233] Langsetmo L, Hanley DA, Prior JC, Barr SI, Anastassiades T, Towheed T, Goltzman D, Morin S, Poliquin S and Kreiger N. Dietary patterns and incident low-trauma fractures in postmenopausal women and men aged >/= 50 y: a population-based cohort study. *Am J Clin Nutr* 2011;93:192-9.

[234] Benetou V, Orfanos P, Feskanich D, Michaelsson K, Pettersson-Kymmer U, Eriksson S, Grodstein F, Wolk A, Bellavia A, Ahmed LA, et al., Fruit and Vegetable Intake and Hip Fracture Incidence in Older Men and Women: The CHANCES Project. *J Bone Miner Res* 2016;31:1743-52.

[235] Langsetmo L, Barr SI, Berger C, Kreiger N, Rahme E, Adachi JD, Papaioannou A, Kaiser SM, Prior JC, Hanley DA, et al., Associations of Protein Intake and Protein Source with Bone Mineral Density and Fracture Risk: A Population-Based Cohort Study. *J Nutr Health Aging* 2015;19:861-8.

[236] Cauley JA. Osteoporosis: fracture epidemiology update 2016. *Curr Opin Rheumatol* 2017;29:150-156.

[237] Kohrt WM, Bloomfield SA, Little KD, Nelson ME and Yingling VR. American College of Sports Medicine Position Stand: physical activity and bone health. *Med Sci Sports Exerc* 2004;36:1985-96.

[238] NSCA, *Health Aspects of Resistance Exercise and Training*, 2004, National Strength and Conditioning Association: Colorado Springs, CO.

[239] Bakker I, Twisk JW, Van Mechelen W, Roos JC and Kemper HC. Ten-year longitudinal relationship between physical activity and lumbar bone mass in (young) adults. *J Bone Miner Res* 2003;18:325-32.

[240] Strope MA, Nigh P, Carter MI, Lin N, Jiang J and Hinton PS. Physical Activity-Associated Bone Loading During Adolescence and Young Adulthood Is Positively Associated With Adult Bone Mineral Density in Men. *Am J Mens Health* 2015;9:442-50.

[241] Daly RM and Bass SL. Lifetime sport and leisure activity participation is associated with greater bone size, quality and strength in older men. *Osteoporos Int* 2006;17:1258-67.

[242] Michaelsson K, Olofsson H, Jensevik K, Larsson S, Mallmin H, Berglund L, Vessby B and Melhus H. Leisure physical activity and the risk of fracture in men. *PLoS Med* 2007;4:e199.

[243] Qu X, Zhang X, Zhai Z, Li H, Liu X, Liu G, Zhu Z, Hao Y and Dai K. Association between physical activity and risk of fracture. *J Bone Miner Res* 2014;29:202-11.

[244] Nilsson M, Sundh D, Ohlsson C, Karlsson M, Mellstrom D and Lorentzon M. Exercise during growth and young adulthood is independently associated with cortical bone size and strength in old Swedish men. *J Bone Miner Res* 2014;29:1795-804.

[245] Allison SJ, Folland JP, Rennie WJ, Summers GD and Brooke-Wavell K. High impact exercise increased femoral neck bone mineral density in older men: a randomised unilateral intervention. *Bone* 2013; 53:321-8.

[246] Kukuljan S, Nowson CA, Sanders KM, Nicholson GC, Seibel MJ, Salmon J and Daly RM. Independent and combined effects of calcium-vitamin D3 and exercise on bone structure and strength in

older men: an 18-month factorial design randomized controlled trial. *J Clin Endocrinol Metab* 2011;96:955-63.

[247] Hinton PS, Nigh P and Thyfault J. Effectiveness of resistance training or jumping-exercise to increase bone mineral density in men with low bone mass: A 12-month randomized, clinical trial. *Bone* 2015;79:203-12.

[248] Hinton PS, Nigh P and Thyfault J. Serum sclerostin decreases following 12months of resistance- or jump-training in men with low bone mass. *Bone* 2017;96:85-90.

[249] Bolam KA, van Uffelen JG and Taaffe DR. The effect of physical exercise on bone density in middle-aged and older men: a systematic review. *Osteoporos Int* 2013;24:2749-62.

[250] Yoon BH, Baek JH, Lee YK, Ha YC and Koo KH. Knowledge on osteoporosis of prescriber according to level of medical institute. *Yonsei Med J* 2014;55:1058-62.

In: An Essential Guide … ISBN: 978-1-53613-331-8
Editors: A. Goodwin and S. Lynch

Chapter 2

WORKING CONDITIONS AND OCCUPATIONAL EXPOSURE AMONG MALE WASTE COLLECTION WORKERS, MECHANICS, AND LORRY DRIVERS IN A MUNICIPAL SERVICE*

Valesca Nunes dos Reis*[1]*, PhD Candidate and Inês Monteiro*[2,†]*, PhD

[1]Faculty of Nursing, University of Campinas, Campinas, Brazil
[2]Work and Health Research Group, Faculty of Nursing, University of Campinas, Campinas – SP, Brazil, and Researcher at the Conselho Nacional de Desenvolvimento Científico e Tecnológico – Brasil - CNPq (National Council of Technology and Scientific Development)

---

* Data from Valesca Nunes dos Reis' doctoral dissertation "Cancer, work environment and prevention: social representations of workers of an urban cleaning service"

† Corresponding Author Email: inesmon@unicamp.br.

ABSTRACT

The aim of this study was to understand the worker's social representation of occupational risks and preventive measures. A qualitative approach was utilised, based on social representation theory – processual approach. The sample was composed by male workers, from a municipal service, responsible for cleaning and conservation of the public area with no permanent contract, in a large city of south eastern region Brazil. The research was approved by the Ethical Board. The interviews were recorded and analyzed according to the social theory representation. 43 men answered a semi-structured interview, performed in the workplace, during their working journey. The majority were black (53.5%), 41 years old or over (65.1%) and married (60.5%). Regarding their function, 18 (41.9%) were garbage collectors, 13 (30.2%) were maintenance mechanics, six (14%) were lorry drivers, three (7%) were public area cleaners and three (7%) were vehicles cleaners. The workers speech was analysed and what emerged were the themes of poor working conditions, unsafe workplace environment and unhealthy working conditions. Regarding the occupational risks we found: chemical risks (chemical product utilized during the work journey, contact with diesel oil, vehicle painting, the use of thinner, gas, degreaser and powder). Concerning to physical risks we found non-ionizing radiation exposure; and the biological risks were the contact with cutting perforating equipment and parts of dead animals. Furthermore, there are other hazards, such as the power relationship among supervisors and the workers, non-compliance with labour legislation and inadequate personal protective equipment. These conditions make these workers subject to situations of occupational vulnerability, requiring measures to improve working conditions and the workplace health promotion. The national and international legislation concerning safety and health at work is not observed and it might lead to unnecessary exposure to chemical and physical agents. Another problem raised by the workers was not having a suitable place for meals during their working journey. The work characteristics, with high physical demand, exposure to cognitive stressors and poor working conditions, might lead to high use of alcohol. The work characteristics indirectly influence the adoption of individual behaviours, which harm their health, increasing the risk of illnesses. The workplace health promotion is essential and occupational health and safety legislation need to be observed, to preserve the health and guarantee a safety and healthy working environment.

Keywords: occupational health, men's health, working conditions, waste collection

Introduction

In the last decades, globalization linked to acute, constant and rapid transformation has instilled the individualistic and fragmented character of human relations, including the ethos of work, that is, the way of being and doing it. In the new productive ideological plan, the exploration and appropriation of the creative, communicational, innovative, flexible, resilient, organizational, cooperative, and resilient capacities and abilities, in the short term and in the absorption of all current information, symbolize the world of work [1]. Highly skilled workers give way to multipurpose and multifunctional workers [2].

Many, if not all, workplaces present risks that might result in illness and physical, psychological and social limitations for workers, and indirectly these damages affect negatively on their families and communities. Identifying and analyzing these risks is the first step towards achieving healthy work environments, established through preventive strategies. It is imperative to overcome the reductionist and erroneous view that the worker is a mere spectator in this process, being delegated to him only the monetary compensation due to unhealthy and dangerous work environments.

Making the worker an active and participatory subject in the process of full recognition of the activity that he/she performs, of the work environment and of the risks involved is an important measure for the transformation and to raise the standards of safety and workers' health protection. However, in order for this translocation to occur in fact, that is, definitive inclusion of workers in the process of discussion, elaboration and democratic decision-making regarding the preservation of their health at work, it is necessary to recognize that, besides the technical and managerial aspects, there are political and economic issues involved in this universe [3].

The National Policy of Men's Health Attention programme was launched in 2008 and supports investments in men's health in Brazil, through the ministry of Health [4].

Waste collection is essential for city maintenance and environmental protection. Usually, it is a low-paid male job, with high physical demand and occupational health and safety risks.

Researchers have described a broad risk and hazards exposure for waste collectors. "Besides the recurrent heavy physical activity, waste collectors are also exposed to bacteria, endotoxins, mould, allergens, particulate matter, irritant inhalants, vehicle exhaustion, atmospheric conditions, noise, and psychomental stress" [5:1].

A study developed by German researchers pointed that "the main duties of waste collectors usually include picking-up waste from its point of production, emptying refuse containers onto trucks, and delivering the waste to disposal and processing facilities" [5:1].

According to the literature, the workers enrolled in waste collection are exposed to fungi [6] (Madsen et al., 2016); diesel particulate matter [7] and mentioned musculoskeletal complaint [5].

A pilot study was developed in Denmark, with a sample of 13 domestic waste collectors workers, during winter, aimed to "(…) examine (their) exposure to airborne inhalable fungal and bacterial species during waste collection, and while seated in the truck cabs (…)" [6:652]. The main result was that "(…) fungal and bacterial species found in high concentrations in personal samples, were also found in truck cabs, but in lower concentrations indicating that fungi and bacteria are transported by the workers into the truck cab" [6:666].

In 2015, approximately 79.9 million tons of urban solid waste was produced, in Brazil, of which 7.3 million tons were not collected and, consequently, had an improper destination. Of this total, 52.6% originated in the Southeast region, with an average production of 107,375 tons per day, and generated around 160,077 direct jobs (71,091 in the public sector and 88,986 in the private sector) in the urban cleaning sector of its counties. Regarding health care waste, 260,063 tons were generated in the same year, of which 180,407 were in the Southeast alone [8].

Every year, waste generation increases worldwide. This scenario generates an increase in the demand for logistics services, infrastructure, human and financial resources. In Brazil, from 2010 to 2014 there was an increase of more than 18% in the number of direct jobs. However, advances in the implementation of an adequate final destination of urban solid waste, health care waste and other wastes do not meet the requirements of Law number 12305, from 2010, on the National Solid Waste Policy. In 2015, 30 million tons of waste were inadequately destined. It is important to highlight that the National Solid Waste Policy makes no explicit reference to workers' health protection strategies [9, 10].

The aim of this study was to identify the profile of the waste collection workers and understand their social representation about occupational risks and preventive measures.

METHODS

Study Design

A qualitative approach was utilized, based on social representation theory – processual approach. The sample was composed of 43 male workers, from a municipal service, responsible for the cleaning and conservation of the public area with no permanent contract, in a large city of the Southeast region, in Brazil. The research was approved by the Ethical Board of the University of Campinas. The written informed consent was signed by all workers before starting the interviews.

The Social Representation Theory as currently widespread in the field of social psychology and sociology of knowledge, was structured in the early 1960s, based on the studies of the French psychologist Serge Moscovici, immortalized in the seminal work entitled "Psychanalyse: Son image et son public." The concept elaborated by Moscovici had its origin in the studies of Émile Durkheim, which first explained it with the denomination collective representations. The term Social Representation constitutes a set of phenomena and their concepts, as well as the elaborated theory to explain them [11, 12]. To anchor a study in social representation theory means to bring into the dimension of the pre-existing representations, that is, the sphere of categories and familiar images, the new, the unknown, the "threatening," so that it can be compared and interpreted. The strange object or idea, when compared to the paradigm of a previously elaborated thought, begins to possess its characteristics and shapes itself in order to fit. Thus, after being classified, named and allocated in a category that historically contains an evaluative dimension, the object gains meaning [11, 13- 14]. According to Jodelet, "anchorage rooted the representation and its object in a network of meanings that allows to situate them in relation to the social values and to give them coherence" [15:38]. It is a process to instrumentalize knowledge, so that when it acquires functional value, it becomes able to interpret characteristics, to understand intentions and motives associated with actions and behaviours, and to manage the context and, therefore, forming opinions [13, 15]. The procedural approach proposes to elucidate the social phenomenon with regard to the processes and conditions involved in the construction, genesis and process of elaboration of the representations. It is the search for the understanding of its generating forces and its constituent elements (images, beliefs, values, information, etc.). The two processes of social representations formation - anchoring and objectification, are strongly valued in this approach. It works with three dimensions: information, attitude and the field of research. As Jodelet points out, "this dimensional analysis is complemented by the research of the principle of coherence that structures the fields of representation: sociocultural organizers, attitudes, normative models or even cognitive schemas" [15:38]. The social representation theory has in Denise Jodelet and Serge Moscovici its main investigators [14, 16 - 17].

The Research Place

The social context of research proposed for conducting the study was a municipal urban cleaning department of a large city, within the Southeast region, with an estimated population of 560,000 inhabitants, of which approximately 31% of them are economically active. The municipal urban cleaning department is an autarchic entity, endowed with legal personality and its own assets, with technical and financial autonomy. The main objective of the department is to promote the collection, transport and storage of solid waste and carcasses of dead animals, as well as to sweep, clean and conserve public places. The entity also has an internal mechanics service for its fleet of vehicles, with a focus on maintenance, painting, renovation and washing, which is also utilised by other municipal authorities. In addition, since 2013, the department has developed a service of castration of dogs and cats, made possible by a bus equipped with surgical and hospital equipment. The department is responsible for managing the collection of household and hospital solid waste, large generators (municipal solid waste exceeding 200 litters or 100 kilograms, waste from workshops and industries, waste, land and other building materials), carcasses of dead animals and other wastes. This activity is organised in 79 collection routes, of which 69 collect household waste exclusively, four collect commercial waste, one special garbage collection (industrial and commercial) and two, hospital waste. The criteria established for the eligibility of the subjects were: age equal to or above 18, not to develop administrative activities and to have a minimum experience of six months in the labour activity. A questionnaire was applied and it was composed of social-demographics characteristics: age, marital status, schooling, kids, and some lifestyle issues, such as tobacco use, alcohol intake and health – Hepatitis B vaccination, physician's examination. The data obtained in the socio-demographic questionnaire were entered in a spreadsheet of Microsoft Excel™ for Mac 2011™ version 14.7. A descriptive analysis was performed, as simple and percentage frequency, with the purpose of characterizing the sample to favour the understanding of the reader about his profile.

RESULTS AND DISCUSSION

Forty-three male workers were enrolled in this research. They answered a semi-structured interview, performed in the workplace, during the work journey.

The average age was 46.1 (SD 10.5) (Table 1) and range from 29 to 68 years. The majority were 41 years old or plus (65.1%), married (60.5%), and more than 50% had completed at least high school (Table 2).

This result regarding age is similar to the German study, where the authors found that "in general, waste collectors represent an aged collective, with the median age at 47.5 years (...) and 66.1% of participants being above 45 years old" [5:3].

Concerning race, 53.5% were black. The mainstream family income was one to 2.99 Brazilian minimum wage, corresponding to approximately US $ 300 – 900 per month.

Regarding their function, 18 (41.9%) were waste collectors, 13 (30.2%) were maintenance mechanics, six (14%) were lorry drivers, three (7%) were public area cleaners and three (7%) were vehicles cleaners. The maintenance vehicles and maintenance mechanics developed their duties in the Department area, and the garbage collectors and lorry drivers developed their duties in different parts of the city, and collect from households and dentists' practices. Public area cleaners develop their duties in specific counties.

Table 1. Distribution of continuous variables according to age, time working for the company and number of hours at work

Variable	n	Average	Standard deviation	Minimum	Q1	Median	Q3	Maximum
Age (years)	43	46.1	10.5	29.0	38.0	43.0	56.0	68.0
Time working for company (years)	43	12.5	8.5	0.50	6.3	14.0	14.8	33.2
Working day - number of hours	43	8.2	1.6	4.0	8.0	8.0	8.0	12.0

A study developed in Greece described the following duties of waste collectors: "(...) collection of household waste and also from the private practices of doctors and dentists" [18: 651], similar to the duties observed in the present study.

Table 2. Workers distribution according to socio-demographic variables

Variable	n	%
Educational status		
Less than 8 years	5	11.6
8 years	8	18.6
High School incomplete	8	18.6
High School	18	41.9
Undergraduate course incomplete	1	2.3
Undergraduate course	3	7.0
Civil status		
Single	9	20.9
Married	26	60.5
Divorced	1	2.3
Living together	7	16.3
Job		
Waste collectors	18	41.9
Maintenance mechanics	13	30.2
Lorry drivers	6	14.0
Public area cleaners	3	7.0
Vehicle cleaner	3	7.0
Type of job contract		
Permanent contract with municipality	35	81.4
Temporary contract	8	18.6
Number of working days/week		
5	11	25.6
6	15	34.9
7	6	14.0
5 days and 6 each 15 days	5	11.6
6 days and 7 each 15 days	2	4.7
12x36 hours	4	9.3
Working time		
Day	38	88.4
Evening/night	3	7.0
Both	2	4.7

The situation in India was more complex, and "the majority of waste workers (64%) were engaged into profession to support family members who were already working. (...). Most of the street sweepers (90%) were employed by a government organisation (...). Waste processors (88.2%) were employed by the private organisations and the remaining 12% work as substitute [19:1193].

Only 9.3% of the workers mentioned sun block use, on a daily bases and some of them use it sometimes (11.6%).

Regarding the type of relationship, in the individual interviews there was a higher participation of statutory workers (69.6%).

The stage of acculturation and environment allowed us to find out that in the functions of weeding, sweeping and waste collection there is a greater presence of temporary contracts, since the workers themselves less value these functions. Whenever possible, those who have a statutory relationship request relocation to the workplace, administrative functions and even to another department of the city hall.

One important aspect to highlight is that 93% of the subjects did not received a physician's examination and the majority have had sick leave (60.5%) (Table 3). The most frequent diseases or problem was depression, low back complaints, cardiac disease, alcoholism, cardiac disease and musculoskeletal complaints.

Fifty five percent of the workers referred alcohol intake (Table 3). This result is higher than the percentage found in the Brazilian National Research, performed in 2013, where it was found that 36.3% of men, aged 18 years or more had drunk alcoholic beverages at least once per week [20].

The majority of the workers (n=40 - 9%) referred not receiving orientation concerning risks prevention, neither about the use of the protective equipment (n=26 - 60.5%).

The only variable associated with family income was the type of food that the worker ate daily and the p-value was 0.0368 (Table 4).

Table 3. Workers distribution according to lifestyle and health characteristics

Tobacco use		
Yes	11	25.6
No	25	58.2
Ex	7	16.3
Alcohol intake		
Yes	24	55.8
No	15	34.9
Ex	4	9.3
Physical activity		
Yes	19	44.2
No	24	55.8
Physical activity out of work (number of days per week)		
1 or 2	9	47.4
3 or 4	7	36.8
5 to 7	3	15.8
Without information n=24		
Sick leave		
Yes	26	60.5
No	17	39.5
Physician's examination		
Yes	3	7.0
No	40	93.0
Type of food		
Vegetables, salad, whole grains and fruits	11	25.6
Vegetables, salad and fruits	8	18.6
Vegetables, salad	17	39.5
Only salad	2	4.6
Only fruits	1	2.3
None of the above	4	9.3

The following occupational risks were found in this study: chemical risks (chemical product utilized during the work journey, contact with diesel oil, vehicle painting, the use of thinner, gas, degreaser and powder). Concerning physical risks we found non-ionizing radiation exposure; and the biological risks were the contact with cutting perforating equipment and parts of dead animals. Furthermore, there are other hazards, such as the power relationship among supervisors and the workers, non-compliance with labour legislation and inadequate personal protective equipment.

The waste collection job involves risks and researchers referred that "hazardous material is often found mixed with (solid waste) and includes discarded medicines, soiled bandages, dead animals, shards, paints and batteries, including sharp items, for example, razor blades, glass culets and metal pieces" about a study developed in the city of Chandigar, India [19:1193].

Table 4. Association between selected variables and family income

Variable	Family income (minimum wage)				p-value
	- 2.99		3 and +		
	n	%	n	%	
Race					0.7385*
Black	15	65.2	8	34.8	
White/'Parda' (not White)	14	70.0	6	30.0	
Tobacco use					0.5703*
Yes/Ex	13	72.2	5	27.8	
No	16	64.0	9	36.0	
Alcohol intake					0.0865**
Yes/Ex	16	57.1	12	42.9	
No	13	86.7	2	13.3	
Sick leave					0.7218*
Yes	17	65.4	9	34.6	
No	12	70.6	5	29.4	
Number of working days/week					0.1117**
5	7	63.6	4	36.4	
6 or 7	17	81.0	4	19.1	
Other categories	5	45.5	6	54.6	
Type of food					0.0368*
Vegetable, salad, fruit, and whole grains	16	84.2	3	15.8	
Other categories	13	54.2	11	45.8	

* P-value - Qui-square test.

** P-value - Fisher's exact test.

Table 5. Association between selected variables and family income

Variable	Type of food				p-value
	Vegetable, salad, fruit and whole grains/Vegetable, salad and fruit		Other categories		
	n	%	n	%	
Age bracket (years)					0.0665*
< 50	16	53.3	14	46.7	
50 or +	3	23.1	10	76.9	
Race					0.1830*
Black	8	34.8	15	65.2	
White/Parda (not White)	11	55.0	9	45.5	
Function					0.0402*
Maintenance mechanics	4	30.8	9	69.2	
Waste collector	6	33.3	12	66.7	
Other categories	9	75.0	3	25.0	
Number of working days/week					0.5188**
5	6	54.6	5	45.5	
6 or 7	10	47.6	11	52.4	
Other categories	3	27.3	8	72.7	

* P-value - Qui-square test.

** P-value - Fisher's exact test.

Hepatitis B virus infection prevention through the vaccination is currently available in many countries. In the present study, the majority of workers (39) had received Hepatitis B vaccination.

One study performed in Greece, in a sample of 208 workers, found that "the prevalence of HBV infection among the municipal waste collectors (…) was 23% [18:653].

The only variable associated with the type of food that the workers' function and the p-value was 0.0402 (Table 5).

Another problem raised by the workers in this research was not having a suitable place for meal during their work journey. The work characteristics, with high physical demand, exposure to cognitive stressors and poor working conditions, can might to high use of alcohol. The work characteristics indirectly influence the adoption of individual behaviours, which harm health, increasing the risk of illness. The national and international legislation concerning to safety and health at work were not observed and this might lead to unnecessary exposure to chemical and physical agents.

One relevant aspect about men's health is raised by a researcher and "efforts to improve the conditions of work, enhance employee participation in decision making, and redesign workplaces to reduce injuries can also improve men's health" [21:729].

However, policy makers and teaching methods need to distance themselves from the normative, regulatory, and even authoritarian character of behaviours and attitudes, so that the translation of knowledge, when it occurs, is truly transformative. In this perspective, approaches that favor collective protection should be prioritised, since collective action has greater breadth, reach and transformation power. Therefore, approaches that combine relational and behavioural interventions achieve better and effective results [22].

Siqueira and colleagues concluded, in a review article about occupational health disparities in the United States, which "local and state initiatives, such as living wage laws and community benefit agreements, as well as multiagency law enforcement contribute to reducing occupational health disparities" [23:557]. The authors give some examples about "the power that organised workers can harness to reduce occupational health disparities" Siqueira [23:568].

Conclusion

The profile of municipal workers enrolled in the process of waste collection were aged workers, married, black and had completed at least high school.

The workers speech was analysed and what emerged were the themes of poor working conditions, unsafe workplace environment and unhealthy work conditions. Regarding the occupational risks we found: chemical risks (chemical product utilized during the work journey, contact with diesel oil, vehicle painting, the use of thinner, gas, degreaser and powder). Concerning physical risks we found non-ionizing radiation exposure; and the biological risks were the contact with cutting perforating equipment and parts of dead animals. Furthermore, there are other hazards, such as the power relationship among supervisors and the workers, non-compliance with labour legislation and inadequate personal protective equipment. These conditions make these workers subject to situations of occupational vulnerability, requiring measures to improve working conditions and the workplace health promotion. The national and international legislation concerning to safety and health at work is not observed and it might lead to unnecessary exposure to chemical and physical agents.

It is a human right, rather than a constitutional one, that workers have access to knowledge about workplace environments free or with reduced risks of diseases and injuries. From this reflection, to overcome not only political and economic obstacles, but also methodological and operational, constitutes a basic element.

Disease prevention and health promotion should therefore be the guiding principles of health and safety legislation and programs at work. Along this line, (re)structuring educational methodologies that promote the access and incorporation of knowledge and, at the same time, empower individuals and groups, is a task already posed, but not yet realised in many realities. There is instrumental knowledge, and in the daily life of relationships, many of those involved are able to fight in a fair and equal way the attempts of submission and devaluation of the worker as being-in-the-world.

Conflict of Interest

The authors declare no potential conflict of interests.

Acknowledgments

The PhD dissertation of the first author received partial support from CAPES – Brazil (Coordenação de Aperfeiçoamento de Pessoal de Nível Superior (CAPES) – Process n. 23038.002221/2014-02.

References

[1] Hennington E, Minayo Gomes C, Machado J, Pena P. Entre o criativo e o precário: reflexões sobre constrangimentos e possibilidades do trabalhador da saúde em tempos líquidos. In: Gomez CM, Machado JMH, Pena PGL (org.). *Saúde do trabalhador na sociedade brasileira contemporânea.* Rio de Janeiro: Fiocruz; 2011. p. 433–52. [Between the creative and the precarious: reflections on constraints and possibilities of the health worker in times liquid. In: Gomez CM, Machado JMH, Pena PGL (org.). *Worker's health in contemporary Brazilian society*].

[2] Druck G, Filgueiras VA. A epidemia da terceirização e a responsabilidade do STF. *Rev Trib Super Trab.* 2014;106–25. [The epidemic of outsourcing and the responsibility of the Federal Supreme Court].

[3] Porto M. *Análise de riscos nos locais de trabalho: conhecer para transformar* [Internet]. INST/CUT; 2000 [Cited 13 May 2017]. Available from: http://pesquisa.bvsalud.org/bvsms/resource/pt/mis-149 [*Risk analysis in the workplace: know to transform*].

[4] Brasil. Secretaria de Atenção a Saúde. *Política Nacional de Atenção a Saúde do Homem.* [Department of Health Care. *National Policy of Men's Health Attention*] Ministério da Saúde. Brasília (DF), 2008; 46p.

[5] Garrido MV, Bittner C, Harth V, Preisser AM. Health status and health-related quality of life of municipal waste collection workers -

a cross-sectional survey. *J Occup Med Toxicol Lond Engl.* 2015;10:22.

[6] Madsen AM, Alwan T, Ørberg A, Urhbrand K, Jørgensen MB. Waste workers' exposure to airbone fungal and bacterial species in the truck cab and during waste collection. *Ann Occup Hyg.* 2016; 60(6):651-68.

[7] Lee K-H, Jung H-J, Park D-U, Ryu S-H, Kim B, Ha K-C et al., Occupational exposure to diesel particulate matter in municipal household waste workers. *Plos One.* 2015; 10(8):e0135229.

[8] Associação Brasileira de Empresas de Limpeza Pública e Resíduos Especiais. *Panorama dos resíduos sólidos no Brasil 2014*. São Paulo: Abrelpe; 2014. [Brazilian Association of Public Cleaning and Special Waste Companies. *Overview of solid waste in Brazil 2014*].

[9] Brasil. Lei nº 12.305, de 2 de agosto de 2010. Institui a Política Nacional de Resíduos Sólidos; altera a Lei no 9.605, de 12 de fevereiro de 1998; e dá outras providências. *DOU.* 3 de agosto de 2010; Seção1:2. [Brazil. Law number 12,305, of August 2, 2010. Institutes the National Policy on Solid Waste; Amends Law No. 9,605 of February 12, 1998; And makes other arrangements. *DOU.* August 3, 2010; Section 1: 2.].

[10] Associação Brasileira de Empresas de Limpeza Pública e Resíduos Especiais. *Panorama dos resíduos sólidos no Brasil 2015* [Internet]. São Paulo: Abrelpe; 2015 [Cited 13 November 2016]. Available from: http;//www.abrelpe.org.br/Panorama/panaroma2015.pdf [*An overview of solid waste in Brazil in 2015*].

[11] Oliveira F, Werba G. Representações sociais. In: Jaques M, Strey M, Bernardes N, Guareschi P, Carlos S, Fonseca T, organizadores. *Psicologia Social Contemporânea*. 21. ed Petrópolis: Vozes; 2013. p. 116–27. [Social representations. In: Jaques M, Strey M, Bernardes N, Guareschi P, Carlos S, Fonseca T. (org). *Contemporary Social Psychology*].

[12] Sá C. *Representações sociais: teoria e pesquisa do núcleo central. Temas Psicol.* 1996;4(3):19–33. [*Social representations: theory and research of the central nucleus*].

[13] Moscovici S. *Representações sociais: investigação em psicologia social.* 3° ed. Petrópolis: Vozes; 2005. [*Social representations: research in social psychology*].

[14] Arruda A. *Teoria das representações sociais e teorias de gênero*. Cad Pesqui [Internet]. 2002 [Cited 15 April 2017]; Available from: http://www.readcube.com/articles/10.1590/S0100-15742002003 00007 [*Theory of social representations and theories of gender*].

[15] Jodelet D. Representação social: um domínio em expansão. In: Jodelet D. (org) *As representações sociais*. Rio de Janeiro: EDUERJ; 2001. p. 17–44. [Social representation: an expanding domain. In: Jodelet D. (org.) *The social representations*].

[16] Ribeiro LP, Antunes-Rocha MI. História, Abordagens, Métodos e Perspectivas da Teoria das Representações Sociais. *Psicol Soc.* 2016;28(2):407–9. [History, Approaches, Methods and Perspectives of Social Representation Theory].

[17] Ferreira SRS, Brum JLR. As representações sociais e suas contribuições no campo da saúde. *Rev Gaúcha Enferm.* 2008; 21(esp.):5. [Social representations and their contributions in the field of health].

[18] Rachiotis G, Papagiannis D, Markas D, Thanasias E, Dounias G, Hadjichristodoulou C. Hepatitis B virus infection and waste collection: prevalence, risk factors, and infection pathway. *Am J Ind Medicine*. 2012; 55:650-55.

[19] Ravindra K, Kaur K, Mor S. Occupational exposure to the municipal solid waste workers in Chandigarh, India. *Waste Management & Research.* 2016;34(11):1192-5.

[20] Instituto Brasileiro de Geografia e Estatística. *Pesquisa Nacional de Saúde 2013. Percepção do estado de saúde, estilos de vida e doenças crônicas.* Rio de Janeiro, 2014. [Brazilian Institute of Statistics and Geography. *Health National Survey 2013. Perception of health status, life styles and chronic diseases*]. [Cited 17 June 2017]. Available from: ftp://ftp.ibge.gov.br/PNS/2013/pns2013.pdf.

[21] Williams DR. The health of men: structured inequalities and opportunities. *Am J Public Health.* 2003;93:724-31.

[22] Goldgruber J, Ahrens D. Effectiveness of workplace health promotion and primary prevention interventions: a review. *J Public Health*. 2010;18(1):75–88.

[23] Siqueira CE, Gaydos M, Monforton C, Slatin C, Borkowski L, Dogley P et al., effects of social, economic, and labor policies on occupational health disparities. *Am J Ind Medicine*. 2014;57:557-72.

Biographical Sketch

Inês Monteiro

Affiliation: University of Campinas

Education: University of Sao Paulo, Ribeirão Preto, PhD.

University of Campinas, Campinas, Brazil, Master degree in Education.

Business Address: Faculty of Nursing. University of Campinas, Campinas, Brazil

Research and Professional Experience: Work, Health and Sustainability; Occupational Health themes; Innovation; Entrepreneurship.

Publications from the Last 3 Years:

Bloch KV, Szklo M, Kuschnir MC, Abreu GA, Barufaldi LA, Klein CH, Vasconcelos M, Da Veiga G, Figueiredo VC, Dias A, Moraes AJP, Souza ALL, Oliveira AMA, Schaan B, Tavares BM, Oliveira CL, Cunha CF, Giannini DT, Belfort DT, Ribas DR, Santos DL, Leon EL, Fujimori EB, Oliveira E, Magliano ER, Silva E, Vasconcelos FA, Azevedo GD, Brunken GS, Dias GM, Correa Filho HR, Monteiro MI, Guimarães IC, Faria Neto JR, Oliveira JS, Carvalho KM, Gonçalves LGO, Santos MM, Muniz PT, Jardim PC, Ferreira PAM, Montenegro

RM, Gurgel RQ, Vianna RP, Vasconcelos SM, da Matta SS, Martins SMM, Goldberg TBL, Silva TLN. The study of cardiovascular risk in adolescents - ERICA: rationale, design and sample characteristics of a national survey examining cardiovascular risk factor profile in Brazilian adolescents. *BMC Public Health* (Online). 2015;15. Available from: http://bmcpublichealth.biomedcentral.com/articles/10.1186/s12889-015-1442-x.

Monteiro I, Taylor P, Iguti AM, Cummins P. Challenges for the workforce development of older workers in Brazil. *Public Policy & Aging Report*. 2015;25:136-8.

Vedovato TG, Monteiro I. Health conditions and factors related to the work ability of teachers. *Industrial Health*. 2014;1:121-8. Available from: http://www.ncbi.nlm.nih.gov/pmc/articles/PMC4202756/

Bordignon M, Monteiro MI. Apparent validity of a questionnaire to assess workplace violence. *Acta Paulista de Enfermagem* (Online). 2015;28:601-8.

Marconato RS, Monteiro MI. Pain, health perception and sleep: impact on the quality of life of firefighters/rescue professionals. *Revista Latino-Americana de Enfermagem* (Online). 2015;23:991-9.

Bordignon M, Monteiro MI.Martins MFSV, Rech CRA, Trindade LL. Oncology nursing professionals' job satisfaction and dissatisfaction in Brazil and Portugal. *Texto & Contexto*. 2015;24:925-33.

Book:

Monteiro I, Iguti AM (org.). *Work, health and sustainability: building citizenship*. 1 ed. Campinas: UnicampFCM, 2016. Available from: ttp://www.bibliotecadigital.unicamp.br/document/?code=71279 &opt=1&lg=en_US/.

In: An Essential Guide … ISBN: 978-1-53613-331-8
Editors: A. Goodwin and S. Lynch

Chapter 3

FACTORS ASSOCIATED WITH PAIN AMONG MALE WORKERS AT THE WHOLESALE MARKET[1]

Stenio Trevisan Manzoli[1], PhD
Aparecida Mari Iguti[2], PhD and Inês Monteiro[3,*], PhD
[1]Prefeitura Municipal de Paulínia – SP, Brazil
[2]Collective's Health Department, Faculty of Medical Sciences, University of Campinas, Brazil
[3]Work and Health Research Group, Faculty of Nursing, University of Campinas, Campinas – SP - Brazil; and Researcher at the Conselho Nacional de Desenvolvimento Científico e Tecnológico – Brasil - CNPq (National Council of Technology and Scientific Development)

---

[1] Data from Stenio Trevisan Manzoli thesis *dissertation Saúde do homem: capacidade para o trabalho e estilo de vida entre trabalhadores de um mercado hortifrutigranjeiro em Campinas-SP* [*Men's health: work ability and life style among workers in a Wholesale Market in Campinas - SP*].

* Corresponding Author Email: inesmon@unicamp.br.

Abstract

The aim of this study is to describe working conditions and health conditions of men from micro and small enterprises in Campinas' Fruit and Vegetables Warehouse Wholesale. The warehouse has in the structure small and micro enterprises, with several employment relationships: formal workers, informal workers (freelancers' porters, owners, permission holders, truck drivers, and temporary workers), rural producers and outsourced workers, in four small free markets and four permanent warehouses and small stores. A cross-sectional study with a sample of 200 male workers was developed. Data collection was performed using the following instruments: Questionnaire with Socio-demographic Data, Lifestyle, Health and Work Aspects - QSETS, elaborated by Monteiro. Data were analysed with the program Statistical Analysis Software - SAS® (version 9.1.3, SAS Institute Inc., Cary, NC, USA, 2002-2003). The level of 5% of statistical significance was adopted. Fisher's exact test and Pearson's Chi-square test were applied to assess the associations among variables. All workers were male, the mean age was 36.8 years (SD 12.1), and ranging from 18 to 77 years. 67% of the respondents were married or had a partner and 72% had children. Regarding exposure to risk factors in the workplace, most workers were exposed to repetitive movements (94.5%), stressful work (75%), pace working to finish tasks (65.5%), prolonged bad posture (90%) and weight lifting (96.5%). For chronic diseases, 19% ingested regular medicine; 32.2% reported some health trouble and 19.5% had medical problems. Workers reported body pain in the last week (23.5%) and in the last six months (40.5%). When comparing their health to people at the same age, 46% believed that was similar. Workers with pain reported worse health compared to others at the same age ($p \leq 0.01$). The workers are exposed to poor working conditions, particularly for physical conditions; there is a higher number of chronic smokers and alcohol's consumers when compared with males in national surveys. Their health status is also worse than general male population, especially for those with pain.

Keywords: occupational health, men's health, working conditions, pain

Introduction

Across a broad range of indicators, men in all socioeconomic groups report poorer health when compared with women, although some high-risk groups include men of low socioeconomic status of all racial/ethnic backgrounds.

Multiple factors contribute to men's elevated health risks, including economic marginality, adverse working conditions and gendered coping responses to stress, each of which can lead to high levels of substance use, other health-damaging behaviours, and an aversion to health-protective behaviours [1:724].

A study conducted in Brazil analysed raw data on national morbidity and mortality, from the health national statistics system in 2001, and it was identified that the current "[…] Brazilian male mortality pattern is similar to other countries. The male death rates are 50% higher than the female ones. Considering the age groups, the highest sex ratio occurred in the age group 20 to 39 years (3 male deaths: 1 female death). Observing the distributions of deaths according to the underlying causes, for both sexes, what draws attention are deaths by diseases of the circulatory system, in first place [...]. Taking into account morbidity, measured by hospital discharges (excluding all related to childbirth/deliverance), there is an equilibrium between the numbers of male and female hospitalizations. There is similarity among the male and female distributions of hospital discharges according to the reason of hospitalization, [except for] the case of external causes and mental and behavioural disorders, with sex ratio of 2.3 and 1.9 male hospital discharges to each female discharge" [2:35].

In the same study, they analysed "the main causes leading to hospitalization [the most prevalent were] diseases of the respiratory system (21.1%), followed by diseases of the circulatory system, infectious diseases, digestive system and lesions" [2:43].

Despite the greater vulnerability and high morbidity and mortality rates, men do not seek, unlike women, primary health care services [3, 4], and usually, entering the health system through outpatient and hospital care of medium and high complexity, which has as a consequence the aggravation of morbidity due to delay in health care and greater cost to the health system [5].

Although policies for workers' health and men's health have been implemented in the last decade in Brazil [5], changes in practice are still poorly observed. Often, due to the difficulty in leaving work to seek care with health professionals (physician or registered nurse, who work in Health Centre) and, in other cases, for lack of awareness of the importance of adopting preventive measures, or participating in workplace health promotion activities.

In a study carried out in the southern region of Brazil, with individuals over 20 years of age, with the objective of identifying the prevalence of low back pain and complaints associated with low back pain, a prevalence of lumbar pain of 4.2% was associated with: “gender, age, marital status, schooling, smoking, body mass index, lying down, carrying weight and performing repetitive movement” [6].

A Brazilian study about men users of the Unified Health Care System (Sistema ùnico de Saúde – SUS, in Portuguese) aged from 20 – 59 years found that the majority considered they had no health problem. “(..) The main reason for failure to seek treatment is no access to services, although both men and women claim the healthcare services receive them adequately. Over 40% of men and almost 30% of women self-medicate” [7:291].

In a study conducted in Japan to assess the prevalence and pain in different occupational groups, associated with occupational and psychosocial risk factors, the pain reported by the workers was related to the working conditions to which they were exposed [3].

Aiming to identify the reasons why some workers remained at work even with non-specific chronic musculoskeletal pain, European researchers from the Netherlands conducted a qualitative study and concluded that personal characteristics and motivation in the workplace were factors that contributed positively to the worker's permanence in their work activities. It is associated to this, the ease of access to health services and rehabilitation interventions and occupational medicine impacting on the sustainable maintenance of the worker in his work environment [4].

There are few current publications that specifically address issues of human health, the impact that work has on health and the presence of work-related pain.

The aim of this study was to describe working conditions and health conditions of men from micro and small enterprises at the Campinas' Fruit and Vegetables Warehouse Wholesale and the factors related to pain.

METHODS

Study Design

A cross-sectional study was developed at the Wholesale Market – CEASA, in Campinas, São Paulo State - Brazil.

Data Collection

200 interviews with CEASA workers were carried out using questionnaires diagnosed symptoms and diseases.

After the authorization of the Ethical Board of the University of Campinas (Unicamp), data collection began in August 2010, and was completed in January 2011. The collections were held at the CEASA-Campinas Hortifrutigranjeiro on alternate days, in order to increase the diversity of sample selection. The companies were randomly selected, in order to maintain the variability of the sample.

The Campinas Supply Center S.A. - CEASA (CEASA - Campinas Hortifrutigranjeiro Warehouse) is the fourth largest in Brazil in terms of sales volume. Because of their characteristics, more than 5,000 workers work daily at CEASA and more than 15,000 people circulate there every day. It has international coverage, receiving products from more than 700 locations in Brazil and around the world, supplying around 500 municipalities. It mainly exports to Latin American countries. It has 570 permission holders, wholesalers and farmers who market their products at CEASA - Campinas, in addition to 835 points of sale of horticultural crops and 504 of flowers and plants. CEASA sells products throughout Brazil, mainly supplying the State of São Paulo and receives products from all MERCOSUL countries, mainly Chile and Argentina [8].

Within the framework of CEASA there are several employment relationships, with registered workers, self-employed (chargers, owners, permission holders, truck drivers, temporary workers), rural producers and outsourced workers.

The men, who were the target of this research, were invited to participate through the CEASA Medical Ambulatory and visit their workplaces, such as the permanent sheds (GP 1, 2, 3 and 4), where there were shops, (MLC, ML1, ML2, ML4), which are large open spaces with landmarks that delimit the place of commercialization of each owner. A brief presentation of the research and its objectives was made, and then spontaneously invited to participate in the research. The free and informed consent form was signed by each participant in two copies and a copy was delivered to them.

Questionnaires

The Socio-demographic, work, health and life style questionnaire - QSETS was developed by Monteiro in 1996, and updated in 2011, containing the following data: demographic variables - age, schooling, time at work, workplace, habits and lifestyle - smoking, alcohol, other drugs, physical activity, risks at work and health issues [9].

Ethical Aspects

Concerning the ethical aspects, the project is in accordance with the determinations of the National Health Council and was submitted and approved by the Ethics Board of the University of Campinas.

Results and Discussion

All the interviewees were male, and the mean age was 36.8 years (SD 12.1), ranging from 18 to 77 years of age. 67% of the interviewees were married or had a partner and 72% had children. Of these, 48.5% had one or two children (table 1).

The interviewees took an average of 52 minutes (SD 0.6) to move to the working environment, ranging from 10 minutes to four hours. The most commonly used means of transportation included: travelling on foot, by bus, car, truck, bicycle and bus.

Table 1. Workers distribution according to socio-demographic characteristics. (n = 200)

Variables	Category	n	%
Age (years)	18 - 29	69	34.5
	30 - 39	53	26.5
	40 - 49	45	22.5
	50 - 59	25	12.5
	≥60	8	4
Civil status	Married / living together	134	67
	Single	49	24.5
	Divorced	13	6.5
	Widow	4	2
Kids	Yes	144	72
	No	56	28
Educational status	< 4 years	8	4
	4 – 7 years	54	27
	8 years	37	18.5
	High school incomplete	23	11.5
	High school incomplete	60	30
	Undergraduation course incomplete	8	4
	Undergraduation course	10	5
Total		200	100

Concerning exposure to risk factors in the work environment, most workers were exposed to repetitive movements (94.5%), stressful work (75%), pressure to finish work on time (65.5%), tiring position (90%) and weightlifting (96.5%) (Table 2).

Table 2. Workers distribution according to self-referred occupational risk factors exposure. (n = 200)

Variables	Categories	n	%
Repetitive movements	Yes	189	94.5
	No	11	5.5
Stressful work	Yes	150	75
	No	50	25
Pressure to finish work on time	Yes	131	65.5
	No	69	34.5
Tiring position	Yes	180	90
	No	20	10
Weightlifting	Yes	193	96.5
	No	7	3.5
Standing while working	Yes	198	99
	No	2	1
Sitting while working	Yes	150	75
	No	50	25
Bending over while working	Yes	187	93.5
	No	13	6.5
Total		200	100

Regarding the characteristics of the work, 49% of the interviewees worked in the Permanent Warehouses (GP) and 51% in the Free Markets (ML).

Approximately 21% of the subjects referred having disease confirmed by physician diagnosis and 63% referred self-reported diseases.

With reference to the use of medicine among the interviewees, 19% referred the use of continuous medication.

In relation to the ingestion of alcoholic beverages, 54% reported to ingest frequently or sporadically, some of these types of drink.

Regarding exposure to risk factors in the workplace, most workers were exposed to repetitive movements (94.5%), stressful work (75%), pace working to finish tasks (65.5%), prolonged bad posture (90%) and weightlifting (96.5%) (Table 2).

For chronic diseases, 19% ingested regular medicine; 32.2% reported some health trouble and 19.5% had medical problems.

Another important aspect is the self-related health and 46% of respondents believed that their health was the same as other people at the same age when compared. This result is lower than the result from national assessment developed in Brazil, in 2013, where 70.3% of men referred their health status as good or very good [10].

Table 3. Workers distribution according to life style and health behavior. (n = 200)

Variable	**Category**	**n**	**%**
Physical activity	Yes	108	54
	No	92	46
Leisure time activity	Yes	195	97.5
	No	5	2.5
Alcohol intake	Yes	108	54
	No	92	46
Tobacco use	Yes	52	26
	No	148	74
Household chores	Yes	93	46.5
	No	107	53.5
Religious beliefs	Yes	137	68.5
	No	63	31.5
Total		200	100

Regarding smoking, 26% were active smokers. The mean time of cigarette use was 14.4 years (SD 10.5), ranging from 90 days to 48 years of use, with an average of 15.9 (SD 7.2), ranging from three to thirty cigarettes per day (Table 3).

The time to go from house to the warehouse took an average of 52 minutes (SD 0.6) ranging from 10 minutes to four hours. The most commonly used means of transportation included hiking, bus, car, truck, bicycle and bus.

About alcoholic beverages, 54% reported to ingest frequently or sporadically some type of drink such as beer, 'pinga' (a type of alcoholic beverage), vodka and whiskey (Table 3).

This percentage is higher than the national assessment, performed in 2013, which has identified that 24% of people aged 18 years or more consumed alcoholic beverage at least one time per week, considering both sexes. The percentage was 36.3% for men [10].

Approximately a quarter (23.5%) of the interviewees reported the presence of pain in the week prior to the interviews and 40.5% in the last six months (Table 3).

The association between pain variables in the last six months with previously selected variables are presented in table 4.

About a quarter (23.5%) of the interviewees reported presence of pain in the week prior to the interviews and 40.5% in the last six months. 46% of respondents believed that their health was the same as other people at the same age when compared.

Workers in the current study reported body pain in the last week (23.5%) and in the last six months (40.5%). When comparing their health to people at the same age, 46% believed that was similar. Workers with pain reported worse health compared to others at the same age ($p \leq 0.01$).

Study performed in France – "The national Health and occupational History survey (...), in subjects aged 20 – 74 years" where pain was self-referred, included "5520 males and 6643 women (...) [and] prevalence was the highest for back pain (35% for males and 37% for females.) The authors emphasized that "for males, the first occupation as a farmer or blue-collar worker was associated with an increased prevalence for most sites of pain, with odds ratios close to 2" [11:331].

Table 4. Association between self-referred pain in the last six months and selected variables. (n = 200)

Pain in the last six months					
	No		Yes		
Age bracket (years)	n	%	n	%	p-value
Up to 30	51	70.8	21	29.2	0.0017£
31 - 40	38	65.5	20	34.5	
> 40	30	42.9	40	57.1	
Kids					0.0002£
Yes	45	80.4	11	19.6	
No	74	51.4	70	48.6	
Compared health					0.0001£
Poor	3	15.0	17	85.0	
Equal	59	64.1	33	35.9	
Bether	57	64.8	31	35.2	
Medicine intake					0.0152£
No	103	63.6	59	36.4	
Yes	16	42.1	22	57.9	
To sleep well after a workday					0.0103£
No	12	38.7	19	61.3	
Yes	107	63.3	62	36.7	
Tiring position at work					0.9617£
No	12	60.0	8	40.0	
Yes	107	59.4	73	40.6	
Total				200	100%

£Pearson's Qui-square test.

Another study preformed in the United States shows that "the prevalence of self-reported low back pain in the previous 3 months among workers (...) was 25.7% in 2010. (...) Female or old workers were at increased risk of experiencing low back pain" [12].

It is important to raise society awareness about the "(...) social invisibility of men's bodies, especially those of men facing social inequalities", as was discussed by Canadian researchers in the literature review about "strategies for dealing with risks and promoting wellness" [13:15].

One of the study limitations is to be cross-sectional, which does not make it possible to identify the cause-effect relationship.

CONCLUSION

200 male workers from the Wholesale Market were interviewed in this cross-sectional study.

The majority was married, had kids and use medicine. 46.5% of them referred to do household chores.

Workers reported body pain in the last week (23.5%) and in the last six months (40.5%). When compared their health to people at the same age, 46% believed that was similar. Workers with pain reported worse health compared to others at the same age.

The workers are exposed to poor working conditions, particularly for physical conditions; there is a higher number of chronic smokers and alcohol's consumers when compared with males in national surveys. Their health status is also worse than general male population, especially for those with pain.

Given that the results analysed showed life and work conditions that are not always favorable to men's health, it is necessary to discuss specific disease prevention and health promotion policies. Bringing men closer to the primary health care services remains a challenge. Such attitudes demand the support from both, the employer and the health professionals, and the workers' awareness.

More detailed studies involving men should be carried out in order to improve working and life conditions, aiming to increase the life expectancy of this genre, as well as reducing public expenditures due to more complexes, long-lasting and low adherence treatments.

Conflict of Interest

The authors declare no potential conflict of interests.

References

[1] Williams, D. R. The health of men: structured inequalities and opportunities. *Am. J. Public Health.* 2003;93:724-31.

[2] Laurenti, R., Jorge, M. H. P. M., Gotlieb SLD. Epidemiological profile of male morbidity and mortality. *Science & Collective Health.* 2005;10(1):35-46. [Cited 13 June 2017]. Available from: http://www.scielo.br/pdf/csc/v10n1/a04v10n1.pdf.

[3] Matsudaira, K., Palmer, K. T., Reading, I. Prevalence and correlates of regional pain and associated disability in Japanese workers. *Occup. Environ. Med.* 2011;68(3):191-6.

[4] de Vries, H. J., Brouwer, S., Groothoff, J. W. Staying at work with chronic nonspecific musculoskeletal pain: a qualitative study of workers' experiences. *BMC Muskuloskelt. Disord.* 2011;12:126.

[5] Brasil. Secretaria de Atenção a Saúde. *Política Nacional de Atenção a Saúde do Homem.* [*Men's Health Attention National Policy*] Ministério da Saúde. Brasília (DF), 2008. [Cited 3 March 2017]. Available from: http://bvsms.saude.gov.br/bvs/publicacoes/politica_nacional_atencao_saude_homem.pdf.

[6] Silva, M. C., Gastal, A., Valle, N. C. J. Dor lombar crônica emu ma população adulta do sul do Brasil: prevalência e fatores associados. *Cad Saúde Pública.* 2004;20(2):377-85. [Chronic low back pain in a Southern Brazilian adult population: prevalence and associated factors. *Reports in Public Health.* 2004;20(2):377-85].

[7] Moura, E. C., Gomes, R., Pereira, G. M. C. Perceptions about men's health in a gender perspective, Brazil, 2014. *Science & Health* Coletiva. 2017;22(1):291-300.

[8] Ceasa. *Central Supply S.A*. [Cited 13 June 2017]. Available from: http://www.ceasacampinas.com.br/novo/Inst_Horti Frutis.asp.

[9] Monteiro, M. I. *Questionário para coleta de dados sociodemográficos, aspectos de saúde, trabalho e estilo de vida* – QSETS. [*Socio-demographic, work, health and life style questionnaire*]. Campinas: Work and Health Research Group, 1996, updated in 2010.

[10] Instituto Brasileiro de Geografia e Estatística. Pesquisa Nacional de Saúde 2013. *Percepção do estado de saúde, estilos de vida e doenças crônicas.* Rio de Janeiro, 2014. [Brazilian Institute of Statistics and Geography. Health National Survey 2013. *Perception of health status, life styles and chronic diseases*]. [Cited 17 June 2017]. Available from: ftp://ftp.ibge.gov.br/PNS/2013/pns2013.pdf.

[11] Leclerc, A., Chastang, J. F., Taiba, R., Pascal, P., Cyr, D., Poluvier, S. et al., Muskulskeletal pain at various anatomical sites and socioeconomic position: results of a national survey. *Rev. Epidemiol. Sante Publique*. 2016;64(5):331-9.

[12] Yang, H., Haldeman, S., Lu, M. L., Baker, D. Low back pain prevalence and related workplace psychossocial risk factors: a study using data from the Nationa Health Interview survey. *J. Manipulative Physiol. Ther*. 2016;39(7):459-72.

[13] Zanchetta, M. S., Maheu, C., Kolisnyk, O., Mohamed, M., Guruge, S., Kinslikh, D. et al., Canadian men's self-management of chronic diseases: a literature analysis of strategies for dealing with risks and promoting wellness. *Am. J. Men's Health*. 2015;1-19.

In: An Essential Guide … ISBN: 978-1-53613-331-8
Editors: A. Goodwin and S. Lynch

Chapter 4

UNRAVELLING DEVALUATION FROM WOMEN'S HEALTH IN INDIA

K. S. Mohindra*[*], *PhD
Subaltern Health, Ottawa, Ontario, Canada

ABSTRACT

India's first prime minister, Jawaharlal Nehru, once claimed that one could "tell the condition of a nation by looking at the status of its women." What would Nehru think of India today? Since his reign, there have been great strides in women's achievements, including rising life expectancy and literacy rates.

However, despite India's growing role as a global economic powerhouse, the low status of women persists, with enormous consequences for the health of girls and women across their life course. In this chapter, I argue that many poor health outcomes of girls and women can be attributed to the low status of women in India. I focus on female *economic* devaluation, specifically dowry - an issue with historical antecedents that has failed to be addressed and perhaps even exacerbated by the entry of the country into the global economy.

[*] Corresponding Author Email: katia.mohindra@gmail.com.

Moreover, the failure to consider this bias in the design of population health interventions may be inadvertently contributing to the devaluing of female lives.

Introduction

India's first prime minister, Jawaharlal Nehru, once claimed that one could 'tell the condition of a nation by looking at the status of its women.' What would Nehru think of India today? Since independence, there have been great strides in the condition of women, including rising female life expectancy and literacy rates. Indian women have been at the forefront of a range of government and private sector roles, from holding public office to taking on leading roles in the banking sector to becoming shining innovators of entrepreneurial activities. There is a strong, vibrant women's movement that has been effectively influencing public policy and negotiating greater space and power for women for more than 50 years (Agnihotri and Mazumdar, 1995; Mathur, 2008). However, in 2011 - despite India's reputation as a global economic powerhouse - the Thomson Reuters Foundation rated India as the fourth most dangerous place in the world for a woman to live, flagging issues such as female feticide and the trafficking of girls and women.

The status of women is intricately interlaced with the health of girls and women; greater autonomy over one's own body and the capacity to convert available resources and opportunities into good health is essential. Persistent anti-female biases produce and exacerbate ill health, including maternal mortality and morbidity, anaemia and nutritional deficiencies, HIV/AIDS and other sexually transmitted diseases, and a range of acute and chronic conditions (Mohindra, 2009; Sen and Östlin, 2007). The poorest health outcomes tend to be concentrated among populations where gender biases intersect with other social stratifications, such as poverty status. Yet, there is a tendency for policy makers to decouple public health policies and interventions from the realities of girls and women, including disregarding social norms with inherent gender biases. While there are a range of factors that influence public health policymaking and action, a key component is the evidence base and knowledge translated by researchers into action. Despite the importance of women's status in the production of health, many epidemiologists and public health researchers tend to inadequately engage with social studies (especially women and gender studies and South Asian studies), often relegating gender to one or two discrete variables of analysis. These types of studies may indicate the presence of gender discrimination as a determinant of health, but will unlikely uncover the complexities of gender and how gender biases can be adequately addressed through population health interventions and public policy.

In this chapter, I argue that many poor health outcomes of girls and women can be attributed to the low status of women in India. I focus on female *economic* devaluation, specifically dowry - an issue with historical antecedents that has failed to be addressed and perhaps even exacerbated by the entry of the country into the global economy. Moreover, the failure to consider this bias in the design of population health interventions may be inadvertently contributing to the devaluing of female lives.

STATUS OF WOMEN

The status of women cannot be isolated from other forms of social, economic and cultural inequalities (CSWI, 1975). Women's status is inextricably linked to her religion, caste[1], and class among other social

[1] The caste system is a social status hierarchy originated within Hinduism, although there is evidence that caste exists among other religious groups in India. Caste is a hereditary, endogamous, usually localised group, having a traditional association with an occupation and a particular position in the hierarchy of castes. At the bottom of the hierarchy are the low-status castes (Scheduled Castes or *Dalits*) and indigenous groups (Scheduled Tribes or *Adivasis*). Historically, *Dalits* and *Adivasis* experienced high levels of discrimination and exploitation by higher caste groups. To correct for this historical oppression, the Government of India adopted a policy of positive discrimination enshrined within the constitution as well as through special legal provisions. Caste hierarchies has historically and continues to intersect with gender hierarchies. Preserving the purity of the ritual order was central to caste practices and was largely accomplished through the subordination of women that is, restricting women's movements, at times through seclusion, and controlling

stratifications, making it difficult to offer sweeping generalisations. Regional patterns in the status of women have also been observed due to diverging marriage and kinship systems, female labour participation and landowning status (Das Gupta, 1987; Dyson and Moore, 1983; Miller, 1981). Furthermore, a woman's status may vary according to the various roles that she plays in her household, within kinship structures and as part of the wider society.

Gender inequality in India is embodied by son preference - a widespread, persistent social norm. Son preference is attributed to a range of factors that privilege sons as an asset, including men's higher earning power and role as providers for aging parents, the continuation of the lineage, male property rights and prominent roles that sons play in religious and cultural rites (Das Gupta, 1987; Vlassoff, 1990; 2013). Conversely, daughters are often viewed as an economic liability, due to exogamous marriage patterns which reduces their value in their natal homes, the marginalisation of women within kinship structures, and limited female ownership rights and decision-making powers. This is compounded by the financially straining dowries that can be impoverishing for many families. Daughters are often viewed as liabilities, a perspective captured widely by social science researchers who have gathered views of community members stating that "Daughters are problems," "Daughters are expenses that go on forever," "When a daughter is born, even a king will become a pauper" (Heyer, 1992; Srinivasan, 2005). Studies have demonstrated not only the existence of a son preference, but also daughter aversion (especially among daughters of higher birth order) - including sex selective abortions and household allocations of resources for medical care and nutrition that are less for daughters, compared to sons (Das Gupta, 1987; Jha et al., 2006). Daughter aversion is most perversely illustrated by

---

their sexuality. These restrictions were placed predominantly on upper caste women as a manner of maintaining caste purity and legitimising and controlling inheritance, notably land. Lower caste and tribal women faced greater social discrimination and had lower economic entitlements, yet had greater autonomy. These dynamics, however, have changed over time due largely to *Sansrkitisation* (in which lower castes emulated practices of upper castes to achieve greater caste prestige), leading to a situation in which low caste and tribal women are generally more impoverished than upper caste women, but no longer in a position of greater autonomy.

the imbalanced, masculine sex ratios (in India, sex ratios are measured by the number of females per 1,000 males). That there are fewer females than males has been demonstrated for over a century, but the child sex ratio (for the population aged 0 to 6 years) has increasingly declined over past decades, with the most recent census 2011 showing 914 girls per 1,000 males (Navaneetham and Dharmalingam, 2011).

Devaluing Women: The Role of Dowry

The *economic* devaluation of girls and women is a multi-factorial, complex issue that cannot be reduced to dowry, but rather an intricate webbing of marriage, gender and property (Agarwal, 1994; Basu, 2009; Kodoth, 2005; Oldenburg, 2002). However, dowry has been viewed by feminists and social reformers as a 'social evil,' an enormous barrier to gender equality and a violation of human rights (Agnihotri, 2003; CSWI, 1975) and will be the focus of the discussion in this chapter.

Dowry is a long standing Indian custom of payments between families upon marriage, specifically flowing from the bride's family to the bridegroom's family. Historically diverse practices were observed across India; 'traditional' dowry occurred predominantly among propertied households in North India and was less common in the South, while bride-price or no payment was observed in the north east (Agarwal, 1994). Where dowries were given, they tended to fall under the woman's control in Southern India, whereas in most parts of northern India, the dowry tended to be subsumed by the in-laws. Some scholars have argued that prior to British colonial rule, dowries operated akin to a social safety net, in which *streedhanam* (female property) was passed down upon marriage under the control of the woman (Oldenburg, 2002; Snehi, 2003). Over time, however, 'modern' dowries have morphed from diverse practices of transferring women's wealth to a singular, pan India approach: women as 'vehicles of capital transfer' (Heyer, 1992).

Modern dowries are marked by three key disturbing trends. First, the costs of modern dowry prices are substantial[2], influencing household savings patterns and intra-household and generational distribution of wealth (Andersen, 2007). Among households with one or more daughters to be married, dowries can even cause destitution (Rao, 1993a). Some peasant households are even forced to mortgage or sell off their land in order to cover dowries. Given that marriage in India is almost universal, households with a daughter face a 'dowry trap,' spurring many families to fulfill dowry obligations that go beyond their means to ensure their daughter's marriage and avoid disgrace (Srinivasan, 2005). In addition to dowry inflation since independence[3], there has been a marked change in the form of modern dowries. Instead of traditional gifts, such as jewellery, saris and small amounts of cash, dowries have shifted to large cash payments, consumer goods (including high-tech items) and real property (Agnihotri, 2003; Ravikant, 1999). During the 1990s, India's economy was liberalised and the country became tightly enmeshed with the global economy. Economic liberalisation led to a flood of newly available goods, leading to a shift in consumer culture. India's neoliberal economic reforms, however, did not benefit everyone equally and many poor and marginalised populations were left with heightened aspirations and limited economic opportunities. Within this context, dowries can be viewed, as a *process of accumulation*, that is the necessary conditions for capital accumulation, restoring or reinforcing power of economic elites (Harvey, 2005).

Second, while dowry was predominantly practiced among certain (usually upper) caste Hindus in Northern India, it has since spread across the country (AIDWA, 2002). Dowry has spread to the south of India, including the state of Kerala which had a history of progressive women's property rights (Kodoth, 2005). Dowry has also spread across castes, classes, religious groups and even among *Adivasis*, India's indigenous groups who tended to have more egalitarian gender norms and practices

---

[2] During the early 1990s, Rao (1993b) estimated dowries to be six times the annual household income in rural areas or 50% of the household's assets.

[3] The magnitude and causes of dowry inflation in India is of considerable debate among economists (cf. Arunachalam and Logan, 2008; Rao, 1993).

(Agnihotri, 2002; Heyer, 1992; Kodoth, 2005; Ramaswamy and Bhukya, 2002; Srinivasan, 2005; Srinivasan and Bedi, 2007). The spreading of dowry from upper to lower castes has been attributed in part to the *sanskitisation*, or emulation of upper caste practices to increase status. Dowry can also be a stepping stone to hypergamy, using marriage towards upward status mobility.

Third, there is evidence of increasing dowry-related crimes, including dowry violence. While dowry itself became illegal in India in 1961, this did little to curb the practice of dowry. Indeed, there have been alarming reports of dowry-related crimes, that include harassment, grave injury and deaths based on dowry demands. Dowry-related violence has been characterised as a form of a 'bargaining instrument,' used to extract additional payments by the husband or his family after the wedding (Bloch and Rao, 2002).

Table 1. Selected Indian laws and international human rights instruments to protect girls and women against dowry-related crimes

Indian Laws	International Human Rights Instruments
Dowry Prohibition Act (1961) Amendment (1984) Amendment (1986)	International Covenant on Civil and Political Rights (1966)
Indian Penal Code § 498 (A) (1983) § 304 (B) (1986)	International Covenant on Economic, Social, and Cultural Rights (1966)
Preconception and Prenatal Diagnostic Act (1994) Amendment (2003) Domestic Violence Act (2005)	Convention on the Elimination of All Forms of Discrimination Against Women (1979)
Prohibition of Child Marriage Act (2006)	Convention on the Rights of the Child (1989)

Source: Basu (2009); Bhave (2007); Ravikant (2000); Shah (2004).

Adopting a legal or human rights perspective, the Indian state has the power to permit or prohibit dowry and dowry-related crimes. A range of powers have been enshrined in Indian laws and international human rights instruments that can be applied to condemn dowry and redress negative and criminal effects related to dowry (Table 1). The giving and receiving of dowry became a crime under *India's Prohibition Act of 1961*; with amendments' to this act expanding the definition of dowry. The more recent Domestic Violence Act (2005) provides a more comprehensive approach to redressing physical harms that may be linked (or not) to dowry; that is, it does circumscribe dowry as the sole cause of domestic violence (Basu, 2009).

How Could Dowry Harm the Health of Girls and Women?

Health implications of dowry vary over the life-course, which will be influenced by a range of factors, including local customs and practices, demographic and epidemiological profiles, poverty levels, as well as gender and caste norms in a particular area. Table 2 identifies six key pathways, delineating the actions that a household may take with respect to dowry, the financial implications undergirding these actions and the potential health implications for girls and women. Key social determinants of health - which are the conditions in which people live and work, influencing their opportunities to be in good health - are included due to their importance in shaping a range of women's health outcomes. In addition, it is important to underscore that since health outcomes are determined through multiple factors and various mechanisms, the proposed pathways are meant to capture the main trajectories fuelled by dowry, that is, dowry should not be viewed as the sole, causal factor of a specific health outcome.

Table 2. Potential financial and health implications of dowry-related acts

Dowry-incited action	Financial implications for households	Health implications for girl/woman
Infanticide/sex selective abortions	Natal household saves money (i.e., no dowry)	Prevent/loss of female life
Neglect of girl child	Natal household prioritises boy children in resource allocation (i.e., food, health care)	Poor nutrition, poor health of girl child(ren)
Child marriage	Natal household saves money (lower dowry; reduce expenses of raising girl child to adulthood)	Early pregnancy & sequelae, multiple unwanted pregnancies, female sterilization, limit reproductive decision-making & education, impinge on rights of child, greater risk for intimate partner violence
Traffic girls	Natal household saves money (i.e., no dowry), makes money (i.e., selling daughter to traffickers)	Dislocation, forced prostitution, enslavement, impingement on rights of child, constrict education, emotional distress, social isolation, harsh working conditions, physical trauma, HIV/AIDS and other sexually transmitted diseases, death
Dowry is given	Natal household, especially poor households, may face downward mobility, impoverishment, household rationing	Poor nutrition and health among higher order girl children
Dowry-related violence	Marital household extracts money, consumer goods	Emotional distress, physical trauma, death

Source: Kuma (2003); Huda (2006); Kodoth (2005); Raj et al., (2010); Raj et al., (2009); Rao (1997); Santhya et al., (2010); Srinivasan and Bedi (2007).

Pathway 1

To prevent having to pay dowry, some families commit female infanticide or have a woman undergo an abortion after sex determination has indicated a female fetus (Diamond-Smith, Luke and McGarvey, 2008; Miller, 1981; Singh, 2013). While female infanticide was historically practiced among certain communities, there is still evidence of the practice today (Diamond-Smith, Luke and McGarvey, 2008; George, 1997; Sahni et al., 2008). More common, however, is the use of sex selective abortions, which has been identified by epidemiologists as the most plausible explanation for India's current low sex ratios at birth (Jha et al., 2006). Economic liberalisation during the 1990s did not lead to a reduction in anti-female bias, but rather an intensification of gender bias, notably natality inequality (Sen, 2003; Srinivasan, 2005). The use of reproductive technologies to eliminate girl children in India was brought to national attention during the early 1980s, but it was with the opening up of the country's markets that families' access to an easy, relatively cheap avenue for sex selection rapidly rose. The commercial advantages of exploiting daughter aversion was assumed by the sex selective technology industry (Arora, 1996; Khanna, 1997). Similar to the dispersal of dowry, the use of sex determining technologies and sex selective abortions have now spread across the country and among communities that did not previously practice infanticide (Jha et al., 2011). For the period of 2001-2005, it was estimated that one female fetus was aborted for every 20 female live births (Navaneetham and Dharmalingam, 2011). Sex selective abortions of girls occur especially after a firstborn girl (Jha et al., 2011; Sahni et al., 2008). Such a strategy ensures the birth of a boy, within the context of the trend towards smaller family sizes (Khanna, 1997). The health consequences are the prevention of or loss of a potential female life. At a population level, sex-selective abortions have led to skewed sex ratios in many parts of the country.

Pathway 2

After the birth of a girl child, the financial distress of having to pay a dowry - especially since the daughter will leave the natal household after marriage - can contribute to neglect of girl children. The link between dowry and neglect of girl children is tenuous since it is much more difficult to isolate dowry from other issues surrounding boy preference and daughter aversion. Furthermore, there has been considerably less research investigating the implications of son preference on living girls compared to issues related to natal mortality (Pande and Malhotra, 2006). However, there is a substantial body of evidence demonstrating the existence of a general phenomenon of daughter neglect (Miller, 1981). Studies have demonstrated the main mechanisms of daughter neglect can be traced to gender biases in household allocation of food, access to health care and preventative health care measures (e.g., immunization), and education (Aurino, 2016; Das Gupta, 1987). Studies have further demonstrated that not all girls are disadvantaged equally, but rather higher birth order girls are more likely to be neglected, that is girls born into families that already have a surviving girl, while girls with brothers and no sisters are more likely to be nurtured (Borooah, 2004; Corsi, Bassani, Kumar, Awasthi et al., 2009; Das Gupta, 1987; Pande and Malhotra, 2006; Singh, 2012). And despite the rise in sex selective abortions of unwanted girls, gender biases in health care have not diminished over time (Singh, 2012).

Pathway 3

Child marriage, which is defined as marriage before the age of 18 years, remains pervasive in many parts of India, especially among the poor. Dowry is a key consideration for earlier marriage, since dowry increases with age of the female, as a strategy to avoid dowry inflation and reduce higher burden of wedding expenses (Kodoth, 2005; Singh, 2010).[4] Child marriage influences multiple social determinants of health, including impinging on child rights, lower levels of educational achievements and constrain female autonomy. Child marriage is also associated with earlier childbearing and other challenges to adolescent reproductive health, such as multiple unwanted pregnancies and constrained reproductive choice,

---

[4] Another key factor influencing child marriage is as a measure of sexual control to ensure the purity and chastity of the girl thereby preserving family honour, a view that is condoned by some religious texts.

which are associated with higher rates of maternal mortality and morbidity (Raj, Saggurti, Balaiah and Silverman, 2009; Sathya et al., 2010). Younger married girls are at heightened risk of intimate partner violence and exposure to HIV/AIDS (Raj, Saggurti, Lawrence, Balaiah, et al., 2010; Sathya et al., 2010).

Pathway 4

In some extreme cases, generally among impoverished families who are unable to pay dowry, families sell their daughters to traffickers (Blanchet, 2005; Ramaswamy and Bhukya, 2002). Girls are usually trafficked at a relatively young age, leading to various factors detrimental to their health, including impinging on their rights, constricting educational opportunities and forced child labour (Huda, 2006). Girls are often trafficked into prostitution and other forced labour. Girls may also be sold or given away as wives[5], generally to areas where there is a shortage of local brides - often areas which are at long geographical distances from their natal homes and of divergent social and cultural contexts from which they were raised. In many cases, especially in rural areas, sold brides are exploited for their labour and are socially isolated (Blanchet, 2005). In some families with multiple daughters, they will pay a dowry and arrange a conventional marriage for their first daughter, then send remaining daughters out as marriage migrants without any obligation for dowry payments (Kaur, 2010). Girls trafficked into sex work face multiple health risks, including vulnerability to HIV/AIDS and other sexually transmitted diseases, gender-based violence, unwanted pregnancies, forced abortions, and a range of mental and emotional health problems (Huda, 2006). Girls who are sold as wives may face harsh, slave-like working conditions and lack adequate social and family networks, including being denied any connection with their natal family.

---

[5] This diverges from the practice of bride-price, which anthropologists suggest is within a ritualised system of exchange between families (Blanchet, 2005).

Pathway 5

Families who pay dowry may face downward mobility, impoverishment or indebtedness, which feeds into the cycle of poverty and ill health found in India (Mohindra, 2009). Poverty is a fundamental cause of ill health and in turn, ill health can cause of exacerbate impoverishment by diminishing potential productive capacities and acquiring financial burdens incurred via health care expenditures. While the consequences of poverty-ill health nexus falls on the entire household, the burdens tend to fall disproportionately on girls and women living in these households.

Pathway 6

Similar to women in other societies, women in India may experience domestic violence for a variety of reasons. Here the interest lies in the specific form of dowry-related violence and harassment. Women with small dowries are especially vulnerable to violence (Rao, 1997; Srinivasan and Bedi, 2007). The most extreme form, so-called 'dowry deaths,' which according to Indian law is attributed to a woman's husband or his family, if a woman dies from unnatural causes within seven years of her wedding and if she had been harassed for dowry by her husband or his family prior to her death. The most typical method of a dowry death is by burning, often dousing the woman in kerosene and then setting her alight, evoking the more popular expression of 'bride burning.' Other methods may also be used, such as poisoning (Kumar, 2003). Pathologists have also documented other methods being used preceding burning, such as poisoning, strangulation, or gunshot wounds (Kumar and Kanth, 2004). It is difficult to ascertain precise epidemiological patterns of dowry-related violence, although there is evidence that a surge of dowry crimes were reported during the 1990s, with dowry-related violence spreading across communities (Kumar and Kanth, 2004).[6]

---

[6] One study identified a 106,000 women (predominantly between the ages of 15 and 34) had died from fire-related deaths in 2001 (Sanghavi, Bhalla and Das, 2009). While this number does not provide a precise estimate of fire-related, dowry-related murders, it does give some indication of the burden of the problem.

POPULATION HEALTH INTERVENTIONS AND ECONOMIC INCENTIVES

Population health interventions include policies or programs - either within or outside of the health sector - that address the underlying causes of ill health embedded in behaviours, contexts and systems of social stratification that increase risk and vulnerability. With respect to improving the health of girls and women, particular efforts are required to design and implement population health interventions that avoid condoning or promoting harmful gender norms. Given India's historical and cultural particularities with respect to gender norms and practices in general and dowry in particular, population health interventions should not exacerbate the economic valuation of girls and women - even unintentionally. Currently, there is a widespread strategy used in public health and international development programs more generally, to incentivise populations, particularly the poor, with money. One of the most widely implemented interventions in India using financial incentives are cash transfers, which is used both within and outside of the health sector.

Conditional cash transfers (CCTs) for health involve the provision of small amounts of cash, typically by governments or charities, once a household or individual has complied with "conditionalities" meant to lead to appropriate behaviour change, ultimately leading to better health and nutrition outcomes (Fernald, Gertler and Neufeld, 2008). CCTs have been implemented as a broader poverty alleviation strategy spearheaded by governments in the global south, most notably in Latin America. Evaluative research of CCTs, such as Mexico's *Oportunidades* program, have demonstrated improvements in maternal child health and educational achievements. Since the late 1990s, when early programs were initiated in Mexico, Brazil and Bangladesh, CCTs have proliferated with strong support from international funding institutions, such as the World Bank and the International Monetary Fund (IMF). It has been argued that CCTs are efficient and are purportedly empowering for women, since money tends to be directly transferred to women and girl children are often targeted for specific health and education goals.

The economist Jayati Ghosh (2011) argues that cash transfers should be viewed as a *complement* to the public provision of services. This is a critical point in India, which lacks a quality, well managed public health care system (Peters, Yazbeck, Sharma, Ramana et al., 2002; Sengupta, 2013). India's health system fails to meet the real needs of the population, there is a lack of equipment and medicine, improper staffing, and is rife with corruption. Furthermore, there is long term, widespread mistrust of public health services (Jeffery & Jeffery, 2010). Maxine Molyneux (2006) has questioned whether CCTs have made contributions to female empowerment in Latin America, pointing out the lack of any discernable effect on intra-household power relations and the redundant, parochial focus of women as mothers and producers of household welfare. CCTs fail to achieve a transformative effect, expanding women's capabilities through changes in oppressive household gender dynamics, providing real opportunities for women to engage in local development strategies for economic regeneration and deepening citizen rights. The lack of research beyond simple impact studies (typically of child outcomes) puts into doubt any tangible benefits for women and evidence of a female empowerment effect (Handl and Spronk, 2015).

The lack of rigorous research investigating the effects of CCTs on women and female empowerment extends to the Indian context. One of the major CCT schemes in India is the *Janani Suraksha Yojana* (JSY), a program launched in 2005 to promote institutional deliveries in order to reduce high levels of home deliveries and maternal deaths.[7] JSY has attracted worldwide attention as the cash transfer program with the largest number of beneficiaries in the world (Lim, Dandona, Hoisington, James et al., 2010). JSY is fully funded by the Government of India, operating under the National Rural Health Mission with the assistance of community health workers, known as Accredited Social Health Activists (ASHAs). The

[7] India has some of the worst maternal health indicators worldwide. Although India has made significant progress in reducing maternal mortality, the maternal mortality ratio remains unacceptably high at 178 per 1000,000 live births according to the Registrar General of India (2013).

program was split into groups: high-focus states, which encompass 18 of the most deprived states and low-focus states, which encompass 10 more developed states. All pregnant women living in a deprived state are eligible for JSY cash incentive, while pregnant women living in developed states are only eligible if they live below the poverty line or belong to a marginalised social group (Scheduled Caste or Scheduled Tribe). Women are supposed to receive the cash benefit immediately at the health care institution or within a week of delivery.

Despite national and international lauding of the JSY program, the evidence base is less than appealing. A large number of eligible women do not use JSY. Moreover, while studies have found that JSY has significantly increased the proportion of women delivering at a facility, they were unable to detect any reduction in maternal mortality (Lim et al., 2010; Powell-Jackson, Mazumdar & Mills, 2015; Randive, Diwan & De Costa, 2013). Qualitative studies have unsurprisingly found poor quality of care being offered for maternity deliveries, deterring some women from using the services and providing women who do use the service with poor quality care, including being maltreated by health care providers (Coffee, 2014; Jeffery & Jeffery, 2010; Vellakkal, Reddy, Gupta, Chandran et al., 2017). Studies have also documented women failing to receive their full allotted cash benefits, due to health service providers capturing rents and administrative errors (Coffee, 2014; Jeffery & Jeffery, 2010; Powell-Jackson, Mazumdar & Mills, 2015). Vellakkal and colleagues (2017) found that it was the ASHA's support services - as opposed to the cash incentives - that was the key enabler of the JSY program, despite ASHAs being poorly paid for their work.

The question of whether CCTs could be aggravating women's low status by perpetuating the norm of attaching an economic value to females has not been systematically explored. Can a program that is based on basic economic theory overcome systematic gender biases, led alone lead to female empowerment? There is evidence that there are gendered economic barriers inadequately considered in the design of JSY, such as women not having a bank account to receive payments[8] (Vellakkal et al., 2017), health providers capturing economic rents, which in turn operates as disincentives to improving women's health outcomes (Coffee, 2014) and unintended consequences, such as incentivising pregnancy (Powell-Jackson, Mazumdar & Mills, 2015). Furthermore, CCTs have failed to invoke one of the cornerstones of transformative programs for women - involving women, especially poor women, themselves in program design and implementation (Molyneux, 2006). Santiago Levy, the Vice President, Inter-American Development Bank and main architect of Mexico's *Progresa/Oportunidades stated that:* "*We could instead transfer income to the poor by subsidizing tortillas, but that would just promote consumption of tortillas*." However, such assumptions neglect the preferences of the poor. In India, the poor tend to prefer receiving direct public provision of essential goods, such as food and fuel to cash (Ghosh, 2011). A survey of women living in Delhi slums reported preferring (almost universally) food rations over cash, due in part to the potential of food price inflations (Parsai, 2011, cited in Ghosh, 2011). Moreover, Indian women have a strong, culturally-rooted preference to deliver at home and mistrust of government health services (Jeffery & Jeffery, 2010), raising obvious questions of whether Indian women want cash incentives for institutional deliveries or would structure the JSY program differently.

CONCLUSION

Monica Das Gupta (2017) recently observed improved trends in female outcomes in parts of Asia due to declines in a culture of devaluing women - issues such as urbanization, education, combined with progressive public policies, have led towards greater gender equality, notably in South Korea. But there are signs that these changes are arising elsewhere, albeit at a slow, often generational pace.

---

[8] In 2014, less than half of Indian women held a bank account.

Improving the health of girls and women in India will need to unravel economic devaluation from womanhood. How is this to be done? Angela Davis powerfully wrote about how enslaved Black women fiercely fought against slavery, with a keen perseverance, leaving a legacy of resistance, self-reliance and sexual equality and nothing less than "standards for a new womanhood" (Davis, 1981). Indian girls and women have and continue to break stereotypes and set standards for a new womanhood by combating infanticide and other forms of gender-based violence, generating their own wealth for their dowries, refusing to pay dowries, challenging excessive and extortive dowry demands, deciding not to marry, and caring for aging parents. Feminist economists have been pointing out the unpaid work done predominantly by females is often uncounted, undervalued and disregarded (Waring, 1988). In India, undervalued work contributions are multiple and include agricultural labour, small enterprises, as well as domestic and child-rearing responsibilities (Srinivasan, 2005).

Research needs to move beyond merely studying the consequences of son preference, towards investigating how son preferences are formed and steps that may be taken to weaken harmful gender norms (Pande and Astone, 2007). Policy interventions will require normative changes and the diffusion of these values (Chung and Das Gupta, 2007). For those of us working in the health sphere, it is imperative that we design and implement population health interventions that shift away from ignoring or confirming negative gender stereotypes and biases to becoming allies in subverting them.

REFERENCES

AIDWA (All India Democratic Women's Association) (2002). *The Practice of Dowry Itself is a Crime, Not Just its Excesses: A Report on the National Workshop on Expanding Dimensions of Dowry*. New Delhi: September 1-2.

Agarwal, B. (1994). *A Field of One's Own: Gender and Land Rights in South Asia.* Cambridge: Cambridge University Press.

Agnihotri, I. (2003). The expanding dimensions of dowry. *Indian Journal of Gender Studies*, 10(2), 307-319.

Agnihotri, I., Mazumdar, V. (1995). Changing terms of political discourse: women's movement in India, 1970s-1990s, *Economic & Political Weekly*, July 22, 1869-1878.

Andersen, S. (2007). The economics of dowry and bride-price. *Journal of Economic Perspectives*, 21(4), 151-174.

Arora, D. (1996). The victimising discourse: sex-determination technologies and policy, *Economic & Political Weekly*, February 17, 420-424.

Arunachalam, R., Logan, T. (2008). Is there dowry inflation in South Asia? *Working Paper 13905*. Cambridge, MA: National Bureau of Economic Research. Available from: http://www.nber.org/papers/w13905.

Aurino, E. (2016). *Do Boys Eat Better than Girls in India? Longitudinal Evidence from Young Lives*. University of Oxford, Oxford: Young Lives.

Basu, S. (2009). Legacies of the Dowry Prohibition Act in India: marriage practices and feminist discourses. In T. Bradley, E. Tomalin & M. Subramaniam (Eds.), *Dowry: Bridging the Gap between Theory and Practice*, London & New York: Zed Books, 177-196.

Bhave, S. (2007). Deterring dowry deaths in India: applying tort law to reverse the economic incentives that fuel the dowry market, *Suffolk University Law Review*, XL (2), 291, 313.

Blanchet, T. (2005). Bangladeshi girls sold as wives in North India. Indian *Journal of Gender Studies*, 12(2&3), 305-334.

Bloch, F., Rao, V. (2002). Terror as a bargaining instrument: a case study of dowry violence in rural India, *The American Economic Review,* 92(4), 1029-1043.

Borooah, V. (2004): Gender bias among children in India in their diet and immunisation against disease. *Social Science & Medicine,* Vol. 58 (9), 1719-1731.

Chung. W., Das Gupta, M. (2007). *Why is Son Preference Declining in South Korea? The Role of Development and Public Policy, and the*

Implications for China and India. Policy Research Working Paper 4373, Washington, DC: World Bank.

Coffee, D. (2014). Costs and Consequences of a Cash Transfer for Hospital Births in a Rural District of Uttar Pradesh, India. *Social Science & Medicine*, 114, 89-96.

Corsi, D., Bassani, D., Kumar, B., Awasthi, S., Jotkar, R., Kaur, N., Jha, P. (2009). Gender inequity and age-appropriate immunization coverage in India from 1992 to 2006. *BMC International Health and Human Rights*, 9(Suppl 1):S3 doi:10.1186/1472-698X-9-S1-S3.

CSWI (Committee on the Status of Women in India) (1975). *Towards Equality. Report of the Committee on the Status of Women in India.* New Delhi: Department of Social Welfare, Government of India.

Davis, A. (1981). *Women, Race and Class*. New York: Random House.

Das Gupta, M., Li, S. (1987). Gender bias in China, South Korea and India 1920-1990: effects of war, famine and fertility decline. *Development and Change*, 30 (1999), 619-652.

Das Gupta, M. (2017). Return of the missing daughters. *Scientific American*, 317(3), 82-85.

Diamond-Smith, N., Luke, N., McGarvey, S. (2008). 'Too many girls, too much dowry': son preference and daughter aversion in rural Tamil Nadu, India. *Culture, Health & Sexuality*, 10(7), 697-708.

Dyson, T., Moore, M. (1983). On kinship structure, female autonomy and demographic behaviour in India. *Population and Development review,* 9(1), 35-60.

Fernald, L., Gertler, P., Neufeld, L. (2008). The importance of cash in conditional cash transfers for child health, growth and development, *Lancet*, 371(9615): 828–837.

George, S. (1997). Female infanticide in Tamil Nadu, India: from recognition back to denial? *Reproductive Health Matters*, 10, 124-132.

Ghosh, J. (2011). Cash transfers as the silver bullet for poverty reduction: a skeptical note. *Economic & Political Weekly*, XLVI(21), 67-71.

Handl, M., Spronk, S. (2015). *With strings attached.* Jacobin, 19.

Harvey, D. (2005). *A Brief History of Neoliberalism.* Oxford University Press, Oxford.

Heyer, J. (1992). The role of dowries and daughters' marriages in the accumulation and distribution of capital in a South Indian community. *Journal of International Development*, 4(4), 419-436.

Huda, S. (2006). Sex trafficking in South Asia. *International Journal of Gynecology and Obstetrics*, 94, 374-381.

Jeffery, P., Jeffery, R. (2010). Only when the boat has started sinking: a maternal death in rural north India. *Social Science & Medicine*, 71 (10), 1711-1718.

Jha, P., Kesler, M., Kumar, R., Ram, F., et al., (2011). Trends in selective abortions of girls in India: analysis of nationally representative birth histories from 1990 to 2005 and census data from 1991 to 2011. *Lancet,* 377, 1921-1928.

Jha, P., Kumar, R., Vasa, P., Dhingra N., et al., (2006). Low male-to-female sex ratio of children born in India: national survey of 1.1 million households. *Lancet,* 367, 211-218.

John, M. (2011). Census 2011: governing populations and the girl child. *Economic & Political Weekly*, XLVI (16), 10-12.

Kaur, R. (2010). Bengali bridal diaspora marriage as a livelihood strategy. *Economic & Political Weekly*, XLV (5), 16-18.

Khanna, S. K. (1997). Traditions and reproductive technology in an urbanizing North Indian village. *Social Science & Medicine*, 44(2), 171-180.

Kodoth, P. (2005). Fostering insecure livelihoods: dowry and female seclusion in left developmental contexts in West Bengal and Kerala, *Economic & Political Weekly* June 18, 2543-2554.

Krishnan, A., Amarchand, R., Byass, P., Pandav, C., N. G., N. (2011). "No one says 'No' to money" – a mixed methods approach for evaluating conditional cash transfer schemes to improve girl children's status in Haryana, India. *International Journal of Equity in Health*, 13, 11.

Kumar, V. (2003). Poisoning deaths in married women. *Journal of Clinical Forensic Medicine,* 11, 2-5.

Kumar, V., Kanth, S. (2004). Bride burning. *Lancet,* 364, 18-19.

Lim, S., Dandona, L., Hoisington, J., James, S., Hogan, M., Gakidou, E. (2010). India's Janani Suraksha Yojana, a conditional cash transfer programme to increase births in health facilities: an impact evaluation. *Lancet*, 375, 2009-2023.

Mathur, K. (2008). Body as space, body as site: bodily integrity and women's empowerment in India, *Economic & Political Weekly*, April 26, 54-63.

Miller, B. (1981). *The Endangered Sex: Neglect of Female Children in Rural North India.* Ithaca: Cornell University Press.

Mohindra, KS. (2009). *Women's Health and Poverty Alleviation in India.* New Delhi: Academic Foundation.

Molyneux, M. (2006). Mothers at the Service of the New Poverty Agenda: Progresa/Oportunidades, Mexico's Conditional Transfer Programme. *Social Policy & Administration*, 40(4), 425-449.

Navaneetham, K., Dharmalingam, A. (2011). Demography and development: preliminary interpretations of the 2011 census. *Economic & Political Weekly*, XLVI (16), 13-17.

Oldenburg, V. (2002). *Dowry Murder: The Imperial Origins of a Cultural Crime.* Oxford: Oxford University Press.

Pande, R., Astone, N. (2007). Explaining son preference in rural India: independent role of structural versus individual factors. *Population Research and Policy Review*, 26, 1-29.

Pande, R., Malhotra, A. (2006). *Son Preference and Daughter Neglect in India: What Happens to Living Girls?* Washington, DC: International Center for Research on Women.

Paul, V. K. (2009). India: conditional cash transfers for in-facility deliveries. *Lancet,* 375, 1943-1944.

Peters DH, Yazbeck AS, Sharma RR, Pritchet, D., Wagstaff, A. (2002). *Better Health Systems for India's Poor: Findings, Analysis, and Options.* Washington, DC: World Bank.

Powell-Jackson, T., Mazumdar, S., Mills, A. (2015). Financial incentives in health: new evidence from India's Janani Suraksha Yojana. *Journal of Health Economics*, 43 (C), 154-169.

Raj, A., Saggurti, N., Balaiah, D., Silverman, J. (2009). Prevalence of child marriage and its effect on fertility and fertility-control outcomes of young women in India: a cross-sectional, observational study. *Lancet,* 373 (9678), 1883-1889.

Raj, A., Saggurti, N., Lawrence, D., Balaiah, D., Silverman, J. (2010). Association between adolescent marriage and marital violence among young adult women in India. *International Journal of Gynecology and Obstetrics*, 110(11), 35-39.

Ramaswamy, G., Bhukya, B. (2002). Lambadas: changing cultural patterns. *Economic & Political Weekly*, April 20, 1497-1499.

Randive, B., Diwan, V., De Costa, A. (2013). India's Conditional Cash Transfer Programme (the JSY) to Promote Institutional Birth: Is There an Association between Institutional Birth Proportion and Maternal Mortality? *PLoS One,* 8(6): e67452. doi:10.1371/journal.pone.0067452.

Ravikant, N. S. (1999). Dowry deaths: proposing a standard for implementation of domestic legislation in accordance with human rights obligations. *Michigan Journal of Gender & Law*, 6, 449-497.

Rao, V. (1993a). The rising price of husbands: a hedonic analysis of dowry increases in rural India. *Journal of Political Economy*, 101(4), 666-677.

Rao, V. (1993b). Dowry 'inflation' in rural India: a statistical investigation. *Population Studies*, 47(2), 283-293.

Rao, V. (1997). Wife-beating in rural South India: a qualitative and econometric analysis. *Social Science & Medicine,* 44(8), 1169-1180.

Sahni, M., Verma, N., Narula, D., Varghese, R. M., et al., (2008). Missing girls in India: infanticide, feticide and made-to-order pregnancies? Insights from hospital-based sex-ratio-at-birth over the last century. *PLoS One*, 3(5), e2224.

Santhya, K. G., Ram, U., Acharya, R, Jejeebhoy, S. J., et al., (2010). Associations between early marriage and young women's marital and reproductive health outcomes: evidence from India, *International Perspectives on Sexual and Reproductive Health* 36(3), 132–139.

Sen, A. (2003). Missing women - revisited. *British Medical Journal*, 327, 1297-1298.

Sen, G., Östlin, P., 2007. Unequal, Unfair, Ineffective and Inefficient-Gender Inequity in Health: Why it Exists and How we Can Change It. *Report to the WHO Commission on Social Determinants of Health.* IIMB & Karolinska Institute.

Sengupta, A. (2003). Universal Health Care in India: Making it Public, Making it a Reality. *Occasional Paper No. 13*. Queens University, Kingston, On: Municipal Services Project.

Shah, M. (2003). Rights under fire: the inadequacy of international human rights instruments in combating dowry murder in India. *Connecticut Journal of International Law*, 19(209), 209-230.

Singh, A. (2012). Gender based within-household inequality in childhood immunization in India: changes over time and across regions. *PLoS One, 7*(4), e35045. doi:10.1371/journal.pone.0035045.

Singh, K. (2013). *Laws and Son Preference in India: A Reality Check.* New Delhi: UNFPA India.

Singh, P., Singh, N. (2017). Confronting gender discrimination in Punjab: evaluating cash transfer schemes. *Economic & Political Weekly*, LII (8), 24-26.

Snehi, Y. (2003). Female infanticide and gender in Punjab: Imperial claims and contemporary discourse. *Economic & Political Weekly*, October 11, 4302-4305.

Srinivasan, S. (2005). Daughters or dowries? The changing nature of dowry practices in South India. *World Development*, 33(4), 593-615.

Srinivasan, S., Bedi, A. S. (2007). Domestic violence and dowry: evidence from a South Indian village. *World Development*, 35(5), 857-880.

Vellakkal, S., Reddy, H., Gupta, A., Chandran, A., Fledderjohann, J., Stuckler, D. (2017). A qualitative study of factors impacting accessing of institutional delivery care in the context of India's cash incentive program. *Social Science & Medicine*, 178, 55-65.

Vlassoff, C. (1990). The value of sons in an Indian village: how widows see it. *Population Studies,* 44(1), 5-20.

Vlassoff, C. (2013). *Gender Equality and Inequality in Rural India: Blessed with a Son.* New York: Palgrave Macmillan.

Waring, M. (1988). *If Women Counted: A New Feminist Economics.* London: Macmillan.

In: An Essential Guide …
Editors: A. Goodwin and S. Lynch
ISBN: 978-1-53613-331-8

Chapter 5

THE USE OF INTRAUTERINE BALLOON TAMPONADE FOR THE MANAGEMENT OF SEVERE POSTPARTUM HAEMORRHAGE

Meliza C. W. Kong [*] ***and William W. K. To*** [+]***, MD***
Department of Obstetrics & Gynaecology
United Christian Hospital, Hong Kong SAR, China

ABSTRACT

Postpartum hemorrhage (PPH) continues to be one of the world's leading causes of maternal mortality. Severe PPH has been variously defined as blood loss between 1000mL to 2000 mL or above. Traditionally, peripartum hysterectomy would be performed in patients with massive PPH as a life-saving rescue procedure in those who failed to respond to uterotonics. Various conservative surgical procedures have been developed in recent years to reduce the need for hysterectomy, including external compression sutures, selective de-vascularization by

---

[*] Corresponding Author: Meliza C. W. Kong, MBChB, MRCOG, FHKAM.
[+] Corresponding Author: William W. K. To, MBBS, MPH, M Phil, MD, FRCOG, FHKAM
Email: towkw@ha.org.hk

surgical ligation or radiological embolization of the uterine and pelvic arteries and intrauterine balloon tamponade (IUBT). Previously, uterine packing has been employed as a conservative procedure to control PPH by direct pressure effects, but has now been replaced by IUBT. Both uterine specific balloons such as the Bakri balloon, BT- catheter or Belfort-Dildy Obstetrical Tamponade System systems as well as non-uterine specific balloons, such as the Sengstaken- Blakemore tube, Rusch balloons, Foley or condom catheters have also been commonly used, and a high success rate of over 80% in general has been reported. Recent data have shown that increasing use of balloon tamponade was associated with a reduction in the need for more invasive procedures such as radiological uterine artery embolization or compression sutures or for peripartum hysterectomy. The good prognostic factors associated with successful IUBT management include early application of the balloon tamponade in the treatment process and the maintenance of a positive tamponade test, while failed "positive tamponade test", coagulopathy, or placenta accreta are associated with high failure rates. There should be vigilant case selection for using IUBT in severe PPH, and in the presence of adverse risk factors, prompt resort to other treatment modalities, or hysterectomy as a savage procedure.

INTRODUCTION

Severe bleeding continues to be one of the leading causes of maternal mortality worldwide. Primary PPH (PPH) is the most common form of major obstetric haemorrhage [1]. The traditional definition of primary PPH is the loss of 500 ml or more of blood from the genital tract within 24 hours of delivery. PPH can be minor (500–1000 ml) or major (more than 1000 ml), and major haemorrhage can be divided into moderate (1000–2000 ml) or severe (more than 2000 ml) [2, 3]. PPH (PPH) accounts for 30.8% of all direct obstetric mortality in Africa and 33.9% of such deaths in Asia [4]. Massive blood loss after delivery can be immediately life-threatening and may rapidly lead to coagulopathy and other systematic complications, with resultant morbidity and risk of maternal mortality. As the prediction of severe PPH on the basis of risk factors is well-known to be unreliable, prevention and treatment of PPH becomes a crucial part of the obstetric management protocol. If conservative measures fail to stop bleeding, surgical treatment becomes necessary. Intrauterine balloon tamponade (IUBT) is now widely accepted an appropriate first-line 'surgical' intervention for most women with severe PPH [2], and high success rates have generally been reported [5, 6]. There is evidence that the increasing use of IUBT has led to a reduction in the incidence of other second-line surgical procedures or peripartum hysterectomy. This article attempts to review the evidence that supports the use of IUBT as a first second-line procedure for the management of severe PPH.

UTERINE GAUZE PACKING – THE ORIGINS OF THE IUBT

The use of uterine tamponade techniques to manage PPH was first mentioned in publications in 1855 [7, 8]. The early methods for tamponade employed uterine packing with cotton gauze. Over the course of time, packing methods with gauze rolls have continued to be used, while other packing tools such as various balloon methods, including the condom, Foley catheter balloon inflation, Sengstaken–Blakemore gastro-intestinal tube, and the Rusch balloon or the Bakri catheter were gradually introduced. Nevertheless, in experienced hands, packing apparently continues to be a safe and effective way of establishing an effective intrauterine tamponade system. In a retrospective series reviewing 87 women who developed PPH after caesarean delivery and were managed by either intrauterine gauze tamponade or B-Lynch suture as second-line therapy, it was found that either method was successful in 52 of these patients with blood loss between 500-700 ml. However, for the other 35 women with blood loss over 700 ml before application of the second-line procedure, additional procedures were needed in 3 of 4 patients who underwent a B-Lynch suture but in none of the 31 patients who had intrauterine gauze tamponade, indicating that the latter performed better in this group of women with more blood loss [9]. In a prospective Chinese study, the outcomes of uterine gauze packing were compared with those of IUBT in the management of PPH during caesarean section, especially for possible increase in puerperal morbidity. Of 318 subjects initially treated by basic management for expected PPH, 99 cases underwent uterine gauze packing and 66 had IUBT as the second-line therapy. The success rates of the two groups were 90.91% and 87.88% respectively. Only one patient in the gauze packing group required resort to hysterectomy. The respective rates of puerperal morbidity were 10.10% and 13.64%, with risk ratio of 0.74 (95% CI 0.32 to 1.72). There were no significant differences between the two groups even after the adjustment for potential confounding factors. The authors concluded that uterine gauze packing was apparently effective in treating PPH during caesarean section without an observable increase in the risk of potential postpartum infection when compared with IUBT [10].

Various Types of IUBT and Results from Case Series

Despite the above findings, in most centres worldwide, tamponade methods using various types of hydrostatic balloon catheter have superseded uterine packing for the control of atonic PPH [11]. Case series have used the Foley catheter [12], Bakri balloon [13], Sengstaken–Blakemore oesophageal catheter [14], condom catheter [15] as well as the urological Rusch balloon [16] (Figure 1).

An early case series on the use of IUBT for control of PPH as well as for acute haemorrhage from the non-puerperal uterus described the use of a Foley catheter inserted into the uterine cavity in 20 patients, and the procedure was completely successful in 17 patients and partially successful in two patients. The authors described the main mechanism of the procedure as the filling the uterine cavity and the cervical canal with enough pressure to cause immediate tamponade between the Foley catheter balloon and the semi-rigid uterine wall. The authors also commented that no special expertise or extraordinary equipment was needed, anesthesia was not required, and no complications attributable to such uterine tamponade were encountered [8].

While the original Bakri balloon was described for placenta praevia [13], such tamponade techniques were apparently also effective in other cases of PPH, such as uterine atony. A prospective observational intervention study was conducted with the Bakri balloon over a 29 month period in Kenya for women diagnosed with PPH (blood loss over 500 mL after vaginal or over 1000 mL after cesarean delivery, and/or hemodynamic changes suggestive of excessive blood loss) unresponsive to standard intervention. Among 58 patients, postpartum bleeding was controlled without further surgical intervention in 55 (95%).

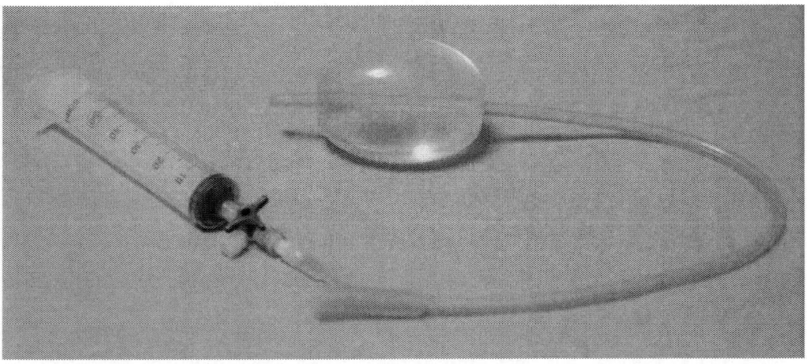

(a)

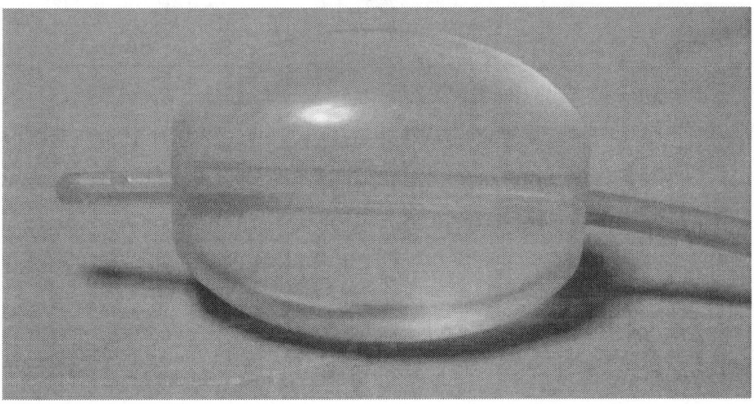

(b)

Figure 1. Example of an intrauterine balloon tamponade device – the Bakri balloon. (a) Two-way catheter for saline infusion into the balloon and drainage from the uterine cavity (b) Protruding end of drainage catheter to allow free drainage from uterine cavity

Among the women with uterine atony, the Bakri balloon successfully controlled PPH in 95%. Two of the three hysterectomies performed were for continued bleeding after placement of the Bakri tamponade balloon.

Four maternal deaths occurred but two were associated with uterine rupture and one with vaginal lacerations, so that only one death was associated with uterine atony. The authors concluded that the Bakri tamponade balloon proved to be an effective adjunct in the management of refractory PPH [17].

Another Finnish series reported 44 women with massive PPH (blood loss >1000 mL) and 6 other women with expected high risk of PPH (blood loss <1000 mL) managed by the Bakri IUBT. The overall success rate was 86% and 7 of the 50 patients needed additional procedures. Among these failures, supra- vaginal uterine amputation or hysterectomy was required in four cases and embolization of the uterine arteries in three cases. The authors concluded that even if IUBT failed, it might provide temporary tamponade and time to prepare for other interventions or transportation from local hospitals to a tertiary centre [18]. In another series of 23 cases of PPH that were unresponsive to medical therapy, the bleeding was controlled in 18 (90%) of 20 patients in whom balloon catheters were properly placed. The other two were deemed to require a hysterectomy, despite proper placement. Technical difficulties led to failure of catheter placement in the remaining three. However, when only cases of uterine atony were analyzed, the success rate was 100% (11/11) [20].

A recent study in Nigeria evaluated the effectiveness of the condom-catheter IUBT in the treatment of women with PPH refractory to first-line treatment. Overall, 203/229 (88.6%) women had successful treatment, which was associated with lower mean blood loss, lower occurrence of blood transfusion, lower intensive care unit admission rates, and lower occurrence of infectious morbidities. A regression model showed that advanced maternal age and caesarean section were associated with lower success rates of the condom-catheter IUBT in comparison with younger maternal age and vaginal delivery [21]. Similar studies have demonstrated a generally high success rates with the condom catheter in developing countries. A review of the effectiveness of IUBT for the treatment and management of PPH in resource-poor settings identified 13 studies of which the condom catheter was used in around 95% of the cases, and was shown to be successful in treating the PPH in 234 out of 241 women [12].

Other reports have focused on the management of placenta praevia/accreta. One series concentrated on evaluating a protocol for conservative measures to treat placenta praevia/accreta over a period of 15 months. Preventive radiological catheterization of the descending aorta was followed by caesarean delivery, use of Affronti endouterine square haemostatic sutures, and placement of an intrauterine Bakri balloon in conjunction with B-Lynch sutures. A total of nine cases were analyzed, and all were successfully treated without resorting to embolization or hysterectomy [22]. In another recent series of 37 patients undergoing caesarean section for placenta praevia/low-lying placenta, it was reported that out of 33 cases in which hysterectomy was not required, 10 (30%) warranted a Sengstaken-Blakemore balloon to control bleeding despite medical treatment. Apparently all of these were successfully treated without additional procedures [23].

As experience accumulates in the use of IUBT, there appears to be a consensus that the success rate for controlling PPH and for avoiding hysterectomy was in general high at around 80-90% [11, 24]. We also reported an overall success rate of 79% over an 18 month period with IUBT alone, which was comparable to the reported rates in the literature [25]. The 2014 Scottish Confidential Audit of Severe Maternal Morbidity report identified 339 women who had an estimated blood loss of 2500 ml or higher. Balloon tamponade was employed in 82 cases and successfully avoided hysterectomy in 75 (91%) women [26], again demonstrating a high success rate that was of the same order as that reported in smaller case series.

Currently, the Bakri balloon, the BT-Catheter (Utah Medical Products, West Midvale, UT, USA), and the Belfort-Dildy Obstetrical Tamponade System (Ebb two-balloon system)(GlenveighMedical, Chattanooga, TN, USA) have been referred to as uterine-specific tamponade balloons [27]. One theoretical advantage of the uterine-specific balloons was that they can conform to the intrauterine cavity once inflated. There may also be a lower expulsion rate or perforation rate. Ultrasound confirmation of the position of the intrauterine balloon has been advocated but this is usually not considered mandatory, as the use of ultrasound has not been shown to lower expulsion rate or other complications (Figures 2, 3). However, both uterine specific and non-specific balloons have in general reported a high success rate despite wide discrepancies in their costs. A recently published Egyptian study attempted to assess the efficacy and safety of condom-loaded Foley's catheter versus Bakri Balloon in the management of primary atonic PPH secondary to vaginal delivery in single blinded randomized controlled trial. It was found that both treatment modalities successfully controlled the primary atonic PPH without statistically significant differences. While the Bakri balloon required shorter time to stop the uterine bleeding than a condom-loaded Foley catheter (9.09 min vs. 11.76 min, $p = 0.042$), there was no difference between both groups regarding postpartum maternal complications, or other vital signs such as urine output or hemoglobin levels. The authors concluded that condom-loaded Foley catheter was as effective as Bakri balloon in the management of primary atonic PPH following vaginal delivery but required a slightly longer time to achieve haemostasis [37]. Apart from this study, there are apparently no other direct head-on comparison data of the efficacy of different intrauterine balloon systems is available in the literature.

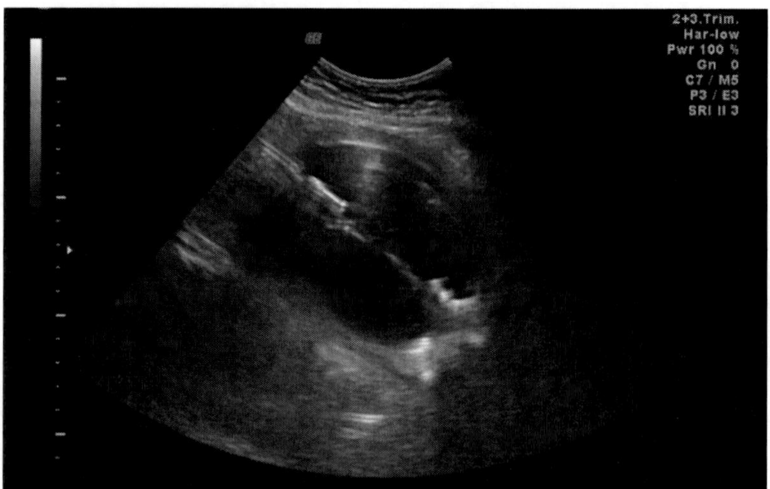

Figure 2. 2D ultrasound showing Bakri balloon within uterine cavity.

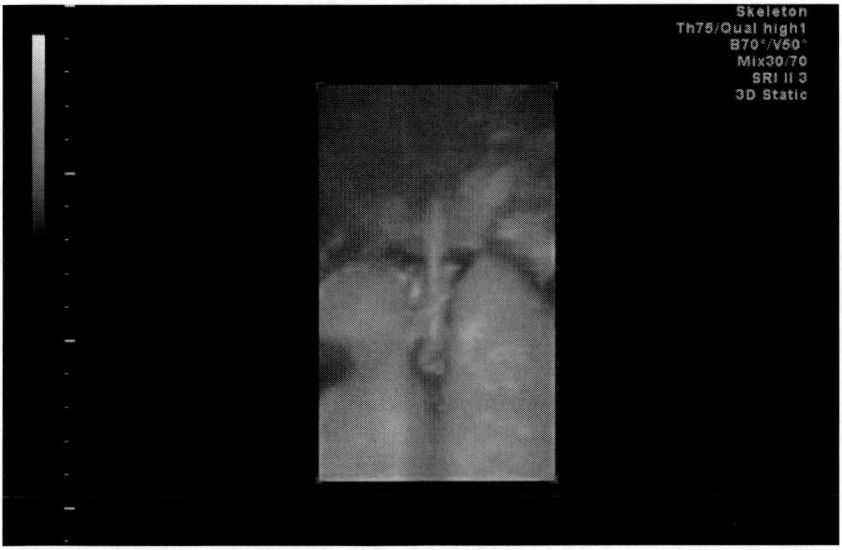

Figure 3. 3D ultrasound showing Bakri balloon within uterine cavity.

THE POSITIVE TAMPONADE TEST

Many of the reports of balloon tamponade describe the procedure as the 'tamponade test' [28, 29]. The first description of such an intervention used a Sengstaken-Blakemore balloon catheter as a diagnostic and therapeutic 'tamponade test' in a series of 16 cases, and it was shown to effectively stop bleeding in 88% (14) of patients for the purpose of avoiding further surgery [19]. The authors remarked that this 'diagnostic' test rapidly identifies patients with PPH that might otherwise warrant a laparotomy. A 'positive test' (control of PPH following inflation of the balloon) indicates that haemostasis has been achieved and further procedures will not be required, whereas a 'negative test' (continued PPH following inflation of the balloon) is an indication to proceed to further procedures including the possible need for peripartum hysterectomy. The concept of balloon tamponade as a 'test' serves to affirm its place as first-line 'surgical' management. [2]. There is no clear evidence on how long the balloon tamponade should be left in place. In most cases, 4–6 hours of tamponade should be adequate to achieve haemostasis and ideally it should be removed during daytime hours, in the presence of appropriate senior staff, in case further intervention is necessary [28]. In a recently published retrospective cohort of 274 women undergoing IUBT, patients who underwent IUBT for 2 to12 hours (75%) were compared with those who underwent IUBT for over 12 hours (25%). The median estimated blood loss after IUBT, the frequencies of blood product transfusion, uterine artery embolization, hysterectomy, and intensive care unit admission were not statistically different between the groups, and this lack of association persisted in multivariable regression analysis. Intrauterine balloon insertion duration over 12 hours was associated with a higher frequency of postpartum fever (27% vs 15%, $p = 0.047$, odds ratio 2.33) which could be related to chorioamnionitis in these cases. The authors concluded that if ongoing haemorrhage had abated, it was reasonable to consider the removal of an intrauterine balloon by 12 hours after its initial placement. [30].

The Use of IUBT with Other Conservative Second-Line Procedures

Various reports have described the use of IUBT concurrently with other conservative techniques. Notably, the successful application of the 'uterine sandwich' using uterine compression sutures in conjunction with the Bakri balloon tamponade has been described in patients with massive haemorrhage due to placenta praevia/accreta [31] as well as to uterine atony[32, 33]. A series of 11 cases with placenta praevia or uterine atony using Hayman sutures combined with the Bakri balloon have also been described [34] with no major complications and a 100% success rate. Another series of 20 cases was published recently, in which the Bakri balloon was used as the treatment of first choice in 20 cases [35]. Of these,

12 were successfully managed with the balloon alone but six warranted the balloon and B-Lynch sutures, while two finally had a hysterectomy.

Comparison of IUBT with Other Second-Line Procedures

The efficacy of intrauterine balloon catheters for the treatment for PPH appears similar to other forms of second-line conservative procedures. In a systematic review of various conservative management modalities for this condition, estimated cumulative outcomes showed success rates of 91% for arterial embolization, 84% for balloon tamponade, 92% for uterine compression sutures, and 85% for iliac artery ligation or uterine de-vascularisation. Nevertheless, the authors commented that balloon tamponade was the least invasive and most rapidly implemented, and that it seemed logical to use it as the first step of management in suitable cases [36]. At present, there are little direct data to compare and evaluate the efficacy of different second-line conservative management modalities for PPH. Understandably, randomized controlled trials would be difficult to carry out in such life-threatening clinical scenarios presenting as a dire emergency. A fair comparison of the different treatment modalities would also be difficult to carry out, as specific treatments may be indicated in specific situations. For instance, IUBT may be particularly indicated for massive PPH after a vaginal delivery, while uterine compression sutures tend to be used (with or without balloon tamponade) after caesarean delivery. Recombinant factor VIIa may be more strongly indicated in the presence of disseminated intravascular coagulation when conventional transfusion of blood products fail to reverse the process, while radiological methods for uterine artery embolization can depend on the availability of expertise of an interventional specialist [25]. It is therefore apparent that the use of these different modalities should be flexible and geared to the aetiology of the PPH and feasible clinical responses tailored to the condition of the patient concerned during different stages of the emergency.

Complications from IUBT

Major complications have been reported following the use of IUBT. Caesarean scar dehiscence has been associated with IUBT placement after a second-trimester dilatation and evacuation [38]. In another case report, ten weeks following application of uterine compression sutures combined with Rusch intrauterine balloon, uterine necrosis ensued and hysterectomy was required [39]. The authors therefore suggested looking out for uterine blanching when applying such balloon/sandwich techniques. Intraluminal pressure has been objectively measured in patients with the Bakri balloon in situ, and it was showed that the intraluminal pressure did not exceed the patient's systolic pressure when tamponade becomes established [40]. Thus, when used alone, the intrauterine balloon is unlikely to give rise to uterine necrosis, but if used in combination with compression sutures, the risks could increase.

Can IUBT Reduce the Need for Peripartum Hysterectomy?

Traditionally, peripartum hysterectomy would be performed in patients with massive PPH as a life-saving procedure in those who failed to respond to uterotonics. However, due to the high morbidity associated with peripartum hysterectomy, various conservative surgical procedures have been developed in the attempt to reduce the need for hysterectomy. IUBT have commonly been incorporated into standard protocols for management of severe PPH as a second-line conservative surgical procedure due to its simplicity and relatively non-invasive nature.

The impact of the increasing use of second-line procedures for the management of severe PPH on peripartum hysterectomy rates have been demonstrated in various studies worldwide. A Korean national wide survey has investigated the trends of peripartum hysterectomy and the utilization of uterine artery embolization from 2005 to 2008, and found that an increase in the performance of UAE from 0.38/1000 to 0.98/1000 deliveries was coupled with a slight decrease in peripartum hysterectomy rates from 1.57 to 1.33/1000 deliveries[41]. The use of second-line therapies including balloon tamponade, uterine compression sutures, pelvic vessel ligation and interventional radiology and Factor VIIa have been shown to be successfully in 74% of PPH patients without the need of peripartum hysterectomy [24]. In addition, in a 5-year cohort from 2006-2011 in a single obstetric centre, it was shown that second-line procedures were used in around 46% of cases of massive PPH, and only 21.4% of the women who received second-line therapies would require rescue hysterectomies. The authors observed a rising trend in the use of second-line therapies, whereas the incidence of rescue hysterectomies and estimated blood loss were found to have concomitantly decreased [42]. Moreover, an analysis on peripartum hysterectomy trends over 4 decades in Dublin showed that the peripartum hysterectomy rates decreased from 0.9/1000 to 0.2/1000 from 1966-1975 to 1996-2005. The authors commented that apart from placenta accreta becoming the increasingly important indication for hysterectomy from 5.4% to 46.5%, hysterectomy for uterine atony has decreased over the decades and was most likely related to the use of conservative management including uterotonics agents, embolization, uterine balloons, compression sutures and devascularisation [43].

Specifically focussing on the impact of introducing the use of balloon tamponade to manage severe PPH that was unresponsive to prostaglandins, a French cohort compared 2 equal periods before and after the introduction of this technique. The success rate with the Bakri balloon was 86%, and the rates of arterial embolization and other conservative surgical procedures decreased from 8.2% and 5.1% in the first period to 2.3% and

1.4%in the second period respectively. While hysterectomy rates decreased non-significantly from 1% to 0.46% in the two periods, the authors commented that intrauterine balloon was an effective strategy for achievement of haemostasis in severe PPH [44]. This was our experience as well. In a large cohort spanning over 16 years, the utilization of uterine balloon tamponade increased from 0% at first to 48.8% in the last 4 years, and the overall percentage that had second-line conservative procedures increased from nil to around 83%. The total mean hysterectomy rates per quadrennium was also observed to fall significantly from around 1/1000 deliveries to 0.6/1000 (p = 0.04) and the peripartum hysterectomy rate also dropped from 40% to 10% in all cases of severe PPH (p = 0.04) [45]. Thus, with the increasing use of IUBT as the first second-line procedure in recent years, both the utilization of other second-line procedures and the need for peripartum hysterectomy were significantly reduced.

Prophylactic Use of IUBT in Placenta Praevia

An Australian study attempted to determine if prophylactic use of a Bakri balloon at cesarean delivery for placenta praevia is associated with a reduced need for additional surgical or pharmacologic measures and less blood loss than usual practices. In a randomized controlled trial, 52 women undergoing caesarean section for placenta praevia were randomly allocated in 1:1 ratio into an intervention arm (prophylactic Bakri balloon immediately following placental delivery) or a control arm (use of any usual surgical/pharmacologic measures to achieve hemostasis). The primary outcomes were the need for further intervention to control bleeding, and the difference between preoperative and postoperative hemoglobin levels. Although fewer women in the intervention group required additional measures to achieve hemostasis during caesarean section, the difference between the groups was not significant (relative risk 0.54; 95% confidence interval (CI) 0.19 to 1.57). The change in hemoglobin level among women in the intervention arm was also similar to that among controls (mean 2.3 g/dL; 95% CI –4.4 to 8.9). The authors concluded that the prophylactic use of a Bakri balloon during Caesarean section for placenta praevia tended to be of benefit, with no evidence of harm or patient dissatisfaction, but the need for additional medical/surgical interventions to control blood loss was not significantly reduced [46].

Use of Balloon Tamponade in Other Settings- Vaginal Haematoma

Severe vaginal lacerations and hematomas can result in serious and life-threatening complications of vaginal delivery. The direct management is usually limited to suturing and vaginal packing with gauze. Bleeding from multiple lacerations is difficult to be controlled by sutures. In these cases, hematoma formation is difficult to be prevented, and when it occurs, its management is usually complex. Vaginal balloon tamponade can be a solution in difficult cases of intractable vaginal haemorrhage or occult vaginal bleeding causing vaginal hematoma. In a series of 4 cases, the authors demonstrated how a self-retaining vaginal balloon tamponade device can be a safe and effective solution. Vaginal balloon tamponade is well tolerated by patients [47]. Similar case reports have also been published elsewhere [48].

Prognostic Factors for Successful IUBT

Despite arguments against the "paradoxical" use of IUBT in uterine atony to expand rather than to contract the uterus, most studies have found that this method was equally effective for managing PPH from uterine atony and placental site bleeding [49, 50]. The timing for insertion of the IUBT appears to be an important prognostic indicator. In a study on the prophylactic use of IUBT in the management of placenta praevia, it was found that fewer women in the Bakri balloon group required additional measures to control bleeding, but the reduction was not statistically significant, so that the value of prophylactic IUBT is still doubtful [46]. In a smaller series of 36 cases of uterine atony, it was found that the Bakri balloon was completely successful for women with bleeding <1000 ml, while the failure rate was as high as 8/20 in those bleeding >1000 ml, and 3/6 in those bleeding > 1500 ml. The authors concluded that the use of the Bakri balloon, if undertaken early, is highly effective for the management of uterine atony [51]. In a French study of 226 cases, the estimated blood loss before IUBT was predictive of IUBT failure with odds ratio 3.2 [52]. While it could be argued that the lower initial blood loss could be due to less brisk bleeding, it was apparent that earlier resort to such second-line surgical procedures would be beneficial in enhancing the success rate.

The manufacturer of some of these balloon systems, e.g., the Bakri, has included disseminated intravascular coagulopathy as one of the contraindications for Bakri balloon management amongst other conditions such as uterine anomalies, arterial bleeding or purulent infection of the genital tract. Coagulopathy would often start to step in as massive bleeding occurred and could be regarded as an inevitable sequel of the uncontrolled PPH. Data in the literature supported the poorer prognosis of patients who developed coagulopathy during the treatment sequence. While it would be difficult to distinguish whether the coagulopathy was the cause or the result of the uncontrolled PPH, once such vicious cycle effects stepped in, the attending obstetrician should be alerted to the high chance of failed management with IUBT. In a series of 137 cases where IUBT was used exclusively for the management of placenta praevia, the failure rate of IUBT in the absence of coagulopathy was 20% while in those with coagulopathy, it was as high as 100% [52]. Other similar studies have also demonstrated that the odds ratio for coagulopathy as a risk factor for IUBT failure was 5.6 [41]. Recent studies have shown the benefits of administration of tranexamic acid in reducing mortality but not hysterectomy rates in women with PPH [53]. While our current protocol did not include the use of tranexamic acid, interestingly a novel attempt to apply anti-fibrinolytic agent topically to the uterine cavity via gauze pack soaked with tranexamic acid wrapped around the balloon was recently described [54]. Whether such methods would be helpful in the presence of coagulopathy would require further studies. A positive tamponade test with the IUBT appeared as a prerequisite for the successful management of PPH [11, 55]. In a series exclusively managing placenta praevia cases, the mean drainage within 1 hr was 60 ml versus 500 ml for the failure cases [41]. Similarly, in a multicentre series, it was observed that bleeding dramatically decreased or stopped after 15 min of balloon insertion in 98.2% of successful cases versus only 15.9% of failure cases [52]. Therefore, failure to cease the bleeding shortly after insertion of IUBT would be a critical prognostic factor.

Whether IUBT management should be attempted in the presence of placenta accreta has been controversial. In a small case series integrating the use of IUBT with compression sutures and endouterine haemostatic sutures for such cases of placenta praevia/accreta has reported a high success rate [22]. However, in a prospective comparison of the use or non-use of IUBT in the management of placenta praevia, it was found that the presence of accreta was associated with high failure rates of 5/6 (83.3%) and the odds ratio for success in the presence of accreta was as low as 0.001 [56]. Due to the high failure rates in the presence of accreta, other studies attempting to evaluate the impact of Bakri balloon on peripartum hysterectomy rates would exclude accreta from the calculations [57].

In conclusion, current data from the literature confirm that IUBT has high success rates in the management of severe PPH, and plays a significant role in the reduction of peripartum hysterectomy. When used with other second-line procedures such as compression sutures, the risk of complications will be expected to increase. Early utilization of the balloon tamponade during the cause of PPH before the occurrence of complications such as coagulopathy should be associated with higher success rates. The presence of adverse prognostic factors such as coagulopathy, placenta accreta and failure to maintain a positive tamponade test should indicate early resort to other management modalities or hysterectomy as a savage procedure.

References

[1] Mousa HA, Blum J, Abou El Senoun G, Shakur H, Alfirevic Z. Treatment for primary PPH. *Cochrane Database Syst Rev* 2014; (2):CD003249.

[2] RCOG. *Prevention and management of PPH.* Green-top Guideline No. 52 Dec 2016.

[3] World Health Organization. *WHO recommendations for the prevention and treatment of PPH.* Geneva: World Health Organization; 2012.

[4] Khan KS, Wojdyla D, Say L, Gülmezoglu AM, Van Look PF. WHO analysis of causes of maternal death: a systematic review. *Lancet* 2006; 367(9516):1066–1074.

[5] Dahlke JD, Mendez-Figueroa H, Maggio LB. Prevention and management of PPH: a comparison of 4 national guidelines. *Obstet Gynecol* 2015; 213: 76.e1-10.

[6] Varatharajan L, Chandraharan E, Sutton J, Lowe V, Arulkumaran S. Outcome of the management of massive PPH using the algorithm "HEMOSTASIS". *Int J Obstet Gynecol* 2011; 113: 152-154.

[7] Ramsbotham FH. *The principles and practice of obstetric medicine and surgery: in reference to the process of parturition*. Philadelphia, PA: Blanchard and Lea; 1855.

[8] Goldrath MH. Uterine tamponade for the control of acute uterine bleeding. *Am J Obstet Gynecol* 1983; 147: 869-72.

[9] Zhao Y, Zhang Y, Li Z. Appropriate second-line therapies for management of severe PPH. *Inter J Gynecol Obstet* 2014; 127: 180–182.

[10] Guo YN, Ma J, Wang XJ, Wang BS. Does uterine gauze packing increase the risk of puerperal morbidity in the management of PPH during caesarean section: a retrospective cohort study. *Int J Clin Exp Med* 2015;8:13740-13747.

[11] Georgiou C. Balloon tamponade in the management of PPH: a review. *Br J Obstet Gynaecol* 2009; 116: 748–757.

[12] Tindell K, Garfinkel R, Abu-Haydar E, Ahn R, Burke TF, Conn K, Eckardt. Uterine balloon tamponade for the treatment of PPH in resource-poor settings: a systematic review. *Br J Obstet Gynaecol* 2013;120: 5–14.

[13] Bakri YN, Amri A, Abdul Jabbar F. Tamponade-balloon for obstetrical bleeding. *Int J Gynaecol Obstet* 2001; 74: 139–142.

[14] Seror J, Allouche C, Elhaik S. Use of Sengstaken-Blakemore tube in massive PPH: a series of 17 cases. *Acta Obstet Gynecol Scand* 2005; 84: 660-4.

[15] Akhter S, Begum MR, Kabir Z, Rashid M, Laila TR, Zabeen F. Use of a condom to control massive PPH. *Med Gen Med* 2003; 5:38.

[16] Keriakos R, Mukhopadhyay A. The use of the Rusch balloon for management of severe PPH. *J Obstet Gynaecol* 2006; 26: 335–8.

[17] Brown H, Okeyo S, Mabeya H, Wilkinson J, Schmitt H. The Bakri tamponade balloon as an adjunct treatment for refractory PPH. *Inter Jo Gynecol Obstet* 2016; 135: 276–280.

[18] Grönvall M, Tikkanen M, Tallberg E, Paavonen J, Stefanovic V. Use of Bakri balloon tamponade in the treatment of PPH: a series of 50 cases from a tertiary teaching hospital. *Acta Obstet Gynecol Scand* 2013; 92: 433–438.

[19] Condous GS, Arulkumaran S. Medical and conservative surgical management of PPH. *J Obstet Gynaecol Can* 2003; 25: 931-936.

[20] Dabelea V, Schultze PM, McDuffie RS Jr. Intrauterine balloon tamponade in the management of PPH. *Am J Perinatol* 2007; 24: 359-64.

[21] Aderoba AK, Olagbuji BN, Akintan AL, Oyeneyin OL, Owa OO, Osaikhuwuomwan JA. Condom-catheter tamponade for the treatment of PPH and factors associated with success: a prospective observational study. *Br J Obstet Gynaecol.* 2017; 124: 1764-1771.

[22] Arduini M, Epicoco G, Clerici G, Bottaccioli E, Arena S, Affronti G. B-Lynch suture, intrauterine balloon, and endouterine hemostatic suture for the management of PPH due to placenta previa accreta. *Int J Gynecol Obstet* 2010; 108: 191-193.

[23] Ishii T, Sawada K, Koyama S, Isobe A, Wakabayashi A, Takiuchi T, Kanagawa T, Tomimatsu T, Ogita K, Kimura T. Balloon tamponade during cesarean section is useful for severe PPH due to placenta previa. *J Obstet Gynaecol Res* 2012; 38: 102-107.

[24] Kayem G, Kurinczuk JJ, Alfirevic A, Spark P, Brocklehurst, P, Knight M. Specific second-line therapies for PPH: a national cohort study. *Br J Obstet Gynaecol* 2011; 118: 856- 864.

[25] Kong MCW, TO WWK. Balloon tamponade for PPH: case series and literature review. *Hong Kong Med J* 2013; 19: 484-490.

[26] Lennox C, Marr L; Reproductive Health Programme, Healthcare Improvement Scotland. *Scottish Confidential Audit of Severe Maternal Morbidity: reducing avoidable harm.* 10th Annual Report. Edinburgh: Healthcare Improvement Scotland; 2014.

[27] Georgiou C. A review of current practice in using Balloon Tamponade Technology in the management of PPH. *Hypertens Res Pregnancy* 2014; 2: 1–10.

[28] Condous GS, Arulkumaran S, Symonds I, Chapman R, Sinha A, Razvi K. The "tamponade test" in the management of massive PPH. *Obstet Gynecol* 2003; 101: 767–772.

[29] Frenzel D, Condous GS, Papageorghiou AT, McWhinney NA. The use of the 'tamponade test' to stop massive obstetric haemorrhage in placenta accreta. *Br J Obstet Gynaecol* 2005;112: 676–677.

[30] Einerson BD, Son M, Schneider P, Fields I, Miller ES. The association between intrauterine balloon tamponade duration and PPH outcomes. *Am J Obstet Gynecol.* 2017; 216:300.e1- e5.

[31] Price N, Whitlaw N, B-Lynch C. Application of the B-Lynch brace suture with associated intrauterine balloon catheter for massive haemorrhage due to placenta accreta following a second trimester miscarriage. *J Obstet Gynaecol* 2006;3: 267-268.

[32] Danso D, Reginald P. Combined B-Lynch suture with intrauterine balloon catheter triumphs over massive PPH. *Br J Obstet Gynaecol* 2002;109: 963.

[33] Nelson WL, O'Brien JM. The uterine sandwich for persistent uterine atony: combining the B-Lynch compression suture and an intrauterine Bakri balloon. *Am J Obstet Gynecol* 2007;196: e9-10.

[34] Yoong W, Ridout A, Memtsa M, Stavroulis A, Aref-Adib M, Ramsay-Marcelle Z, Fakokunde A. Application of uterine compression suture in association with intrauterine balloon tamponade (uterine sandwich) for PPH. *Acta Obstet Gynecol Scand* 2012;91:147-51.

[35] Diemert A, Ortmeyer G, Hollwitz B, Lotz M, Somville T, Glosemeyer P, Diehl W, Hecher K. The combination of intrauterine balloon tamponade and the B-Lynch procedure for the treatment of severe PPH. *Am J Obstet Gynecol* 2012; 206: 65.e1-4.

[36] Doumouchtsis SK, Papageorghiou AT, Vernier C, Arulkumaran S. Management of PPH by uterine balloon tamponade: prospective evaluation of effectiveness. *Acta Obstet Gynecol Scand* 2008;87: 849-855.

[37] Darwish AM, Abdallah MM, Shaaban OM, Ali MK, Khalaf M, Sabra AMA. Bakri balloon versus condom-loaded Foley's catheter for treatment of atonic PPH secondary to vaginal delivery: a randomized controlled trial. *J Matern Fetal Neonatal Med* 2017; epub July. DOI: 10.1080/14767058.2017.1297407.

[38] Soon R, Aeby T, Kaneshiro B. Cesarean scar dehiscence associated with intrauterine balloon tamponade placement after a second trimester dilatation and evacuation. *Hawaii Med J* 2011; 70: 137-138.

[39] Lodhi W, Golara M, Karangaokar V, Yoong W. Uterine necrosis following application of combined uterine compression suture with intrauterine balloon tamponade. *J Obstet Gynaecol* 2012;32: 30-1.

[40] Georgiou C. Intraluminal pressure readings during the establishment of a positive "tamponade test" in the management of PPH. *Br J Obstet Gynaecol* 2009;117: 295-303.

[41] Cho GJ, Kim LY, Hong HR, et al. Trends in the rates of peripartum hysterectomy and uterine artery embolization. *PLoS One.* 2013; 8(4): e60512.

[42] Chan LL, Lo TK, Lau WL, Lau S, Law B, Tsang HH, Leung WC. Use of second line therapies for management of massive primary PPH. *Int J Obstet Gynecol* 2013; 122; 238-243.

[43] Flood KM, Sid S, Geary M, Robson M, Fitzpatrick C, Malone FD. Changing trends in peripartum hysterectomy over the last 4 decades. *Am J Obstet Gynecol* 2009; 200: 632 e1-e6.

[44] Laas E, Bui C, Popowski T, Mbaku OM, Rozenberg P. Trends in the rate of invasive procedures after the addition of the intrauterine tamponade test to a protocol for management of severe PPH. *Am J Obstet Gynecol* 2012; 207: 281 e1-7.

[45] Kong CW, To WWK. Trends in conservative procedures and peripartum hysterectomy rates in severe PPH. *J Matern Fetal Neonatal Med 2017,* ePub July 2017 DOI 10.1080/14767058.2017. 1357169.

[46] Beckmann MM, Chaplin J. Bakri balloon during cesarean delivery for placenta previa. *Inter J Gynecol Obstet* 2014; 124: 118–122.

[47] Ghirardini G, Alboni C, Mabrouk M. Use of Balloon Tamponade in Management of Severe Postprtum Vaginal Haemorrhage and Vaginal Hematoma: A Case Series. *Gynecol Obstet Invest* 2012; 74: 320–323.

[48] Atilgan R, Ozkan ZS, Orak U, Baspinar M. Complete tamponade system for management of severe postpartum vaginal haemorrhage due to uterine atony. *Br Med J Case Rep* 2014. doi:10.1136/bcr-2014-205872.

[49] Olsen R, Reisner DP, Benedetti TJ, Dunsmoor-Su RF. Bakri balloon effectiveness for PPH: a "real world experience". *J Matern Fetal Neonatal Med* 2013; 26:1720-1723.

[50] Son M, Einerson B, Schneider P, Fields IC, Grobman WA, Miller ES. Is there an association between indication for intrauterine balloon tamponade and balloon failure? *Am J Perinatol* 2017; 34:164-168.

[51] Vintejoux E, Ulrich D, Mousty E, Masia F, Mares P, de Tayrac R, Letouzey V. Success factors for bakri balloon usage secondary to

uterine atony: a retrospective multicentre study. *Aust NZ J Obstet Gynaecol* 2015; 55: 572-577.

[52] Revert M, Cottenet J, Raynal P, Cibot E, Quantin C, Rosenberg P. Intrauterine balloon tamponade for management of severe PPH in a perinatal network: a prospective study. *Br J Obstet Gynaecol* 2017; 124:1255-1262.

[53] WOMAN Trail collaborators. Effect of early tranexamic acid administration on mortality, hysterectomy, and other morbidities in women with PPH (WOMAN): an international randomized, double blind, placebo-controlled trial. *Lancet* 2017; 389:2105-2116.

[54] Kinugasa M, Tamai H, Miyake M, Shimizu T. Uterine balloon tamponade in combination with topical administration of tranexamic acid for management of PPH. *Case Reports in Obstet Gynecol* 2015; 2015:195036.

[55] Arulkumaran S, Condus G. The tamponade test in the management of massive PPH. *Obstet Gyneco* 2003; 102: 641-642.

[56] Lo A, St Marie P, Yadav P, Belisle E, Markenson G. The impact of Bakri balloon tamponade on the rate of postpartum hysterectomy for uterine atony. *J Matern Fetal Neonatal Med* 2016; 29:1-4.

[57] Maher MA, Abdelaziz A. Comparison between two management protocols for PPH during caesarean section in placenta previa: balloon protocol versus non-balloon protocol. *J Obstet Gynecol Res* 2017; 43:447-455.

In: An Essential Guide … ISBN: 978-1-53613-331-8
Editors: A. Goodwin and S. Lynch

Chapter 6

THE PHARMACOKINETICS OF TERATOGENESIS

Charles Savona-Ventura[1,*] and Yvonne Savona-Ventura[2]
[1] Department of Obstetrics and Gynaecology
[2] Department of Pharmacy, Faculty of Medicine and Surgery,
University of Malta, Msida, Malta

ABSTRACT

The development of congenital malformations is often associated with teratogenesis brought on by adverse conditions within the *millieur interieur* of the developing embryo. These adverse conditions can range from infective organisms to chemical substances or physical damage exerted onto the developing cells. The teratogenic process is generally considered to give rise to structural abnormalities. The pharmacokinetic processes have to be seen in the perspective of maternal and fetal lethal dose parameters.

* Corresponding Author Email: charles.savona-ventura@um.edu.mt.

INTRODUCTION

The latter part of the twentieth century brought about an increasing realization that exogenous factors could adversely affect the developing fetus. The experiences following the development of nuclear warfare, the rubella-malformations association and the thalidomide catastrophe emphasized the potential adverse roles played by exogenous factors on the developing fetus [1, 2]. A wide variety of physical, biological and chemical exogenous factors have since been identified as being teratotoxic and thus interfering with the development of the fetus at various stages of its development.

Fetal development can be broadly viewed into three phases. The first phase is that referred to as the Germinal Period lasting from conception up to day 16 of development. This is the phase when blastogenesis is taking place starting with the production of the zygote at conception followed by simple mitotic cell division producing by day 4 a structure resembling a hollow ball of about 60-70 cells known as the blastocyst or blastula. At day 6, the blastocyst reaches the uterine cavity and initiates implantation into the secretory endometrium a process that takes a few days to complete and which process initiates the development of the placenta. During the pre-implantation phase, the demand for energy required for the increased synthesis of macromolecules serving as the building blocks of cellular reproduction is obtained from the secretions provided by the Fallopian tube cells and endometrial glands. The zygote is thus washed by maternal extracellular fluid and obtains its requirements from the secretions. Once implantation initiates, the nutritional demands are met by substances in maternal blood. The developing zygote initially exhibits a preference for oxidizable energy-providing substrates such as non-essential amino acids, pyruvate and glutamine. There is subsequently a biochemical shift during preimplantation development with the energy metabolism shifting from one primarily based on aerobic metabolism to one based on aerobic glycolysis and oxidative metabolism. Glucose and essential amino acids thus become increasingly more important with advancing development [3]. Alterations in the metabolic processes, as happens in the uncontrolled diabetic, have also been shown in animal studies to predispose towards damage to the zygote and a higher risk of resorption of the developing zygotes [4]. The rapidly dividing cells of the zygote will absorb and assimilate all substances having the capacity of diffusion following the principles of cell membrane transfer. The presence of teratotoxic substances at this stage will interfere with cellular development causing damage to the developing blastocyst. This damage may be repaired or may be sufficiently significant to result in cellular death and resorption before implantation or expulsion during the subsequent menstruation after implantation. Despite the fact that the pre-implantation zygote in not yet in direct contact with the maternal blood supply, it is still able to sense and react to the biochemical environment and through the capacity of developmental plasticity and epigenetic mechanisms initiate adaptive processes that may result in long-term consequences [5]. The proportion of human conceptions that terminate into resorbed or early expulsion zygotes is not known but animal studies suggest that about 60% of zygotes fail to implant successfully.

Following implantation, the zygote initiates the process of embryogenesis, a period of marked structural development and the development of a fetal support system including the placenta, umbilical cord and amniotic sac. Any serious error of development during embryogenesis will generally result in a spontaneous miscarriage. However, if the developmental error is not lethal, the process at this stage of development can result in a morphological malformation. This process can be adversely influenced by various physical, biological and chemical exogenous or endogenous teratogenic factors (Figure 1).

About 15-20 percent of human pregnancies are estimated to end in a spontaneous miscarriage. While a proportion of these may be the result of genetic factors, a significant proportion will be due to teratotoxic influences during the embryogenic period of development. Alterations in the metabolic processes, as happens in the uncontrolled diabetic, have also been shown in animal studies to predispose towards a higher risk of spontaneous miscarriages and congenital anomalies, emphasizing the need of ideal preconceptional metabolic control in known diabetics to improve fertility and reduce the risk of miscarriage [4].

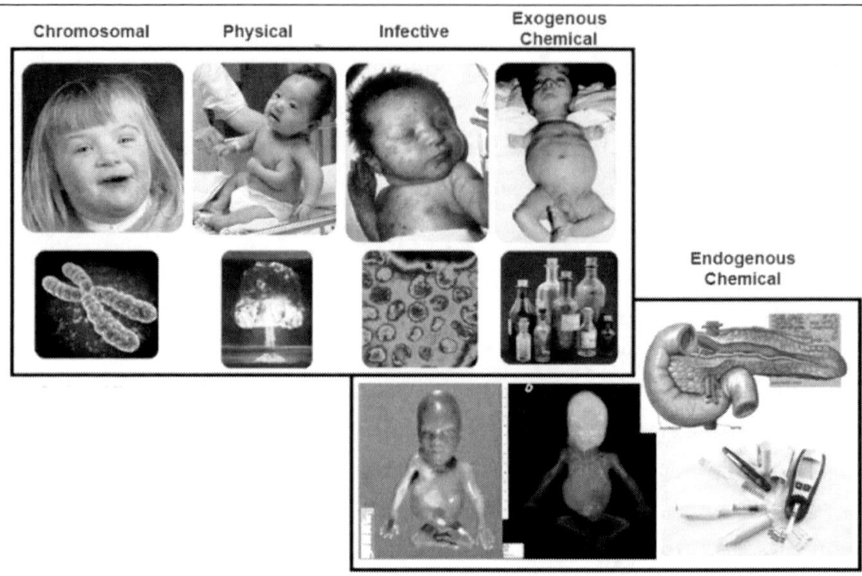

Exogenous

- Physical: Temperature changes, lack of oxygen, mechanical influences, ultrasound, ionizing radiation, electric current
- Chemical: Medicaments, poisons
- Biological: Viruses, bacteria, parasites

Endogenous

- Maternal body factors: Metabolic products, hormones, autoimmune antibodies [e.g., SLE]
- Nutritional states: Vitamin deficiency, nutritional deficiencies

Figure 1. Types of teratogens.

The effects of teratotoxic factors on the developing embryo will depend on the stage of development the embryo has reached at its time of exposure and on the duration period the embryo is exposed to the agent. This relationship was best demonstrated in the effects reported after the administration of thalidomide in the late 1950s and early 1960s. Thalidomide, administered as an antiemetic to treat morning sickness in pregnant women, caused severe birth defects involving the skeleton and soft tissue organs including heart, kidney, and gastrointestinal tract giving rise to what has been termed as the thalidomide embryopathy or syndrome [6]. The administration time-determined effects of thalidomide (Figure 2) were demonstrated in the original published observations by E. Nowack in 1965 [7]. Teratotoxic agents will thus affect the organs under development at the time or period of administration (Figure 3).

The third phase of development is referred to as the fetal phase when the development concentrates on fetal growth and organ differentiation. With increasing differentiation of the organs, the sensitivity of the developing fetus to teratotoxic agents diminishes. However, fetal organ function differs from that of the infant or adult, and potential toxicological and pharmacological effects are dependent on the degree of morphological differentiation of the organs and also on the degree of enzyme maturation affecting acetylation and conjugation processes. The concept of teratogenesis was widened from the narrow confines of structural abnormalities to include adult-onset carcinogenesis following the identification in 1956 of the role of x-ray radiation on the subsequent development of childhood leukemia [8], and the association in the early 1970s between antenatal use of diethylstilboestrol and vaginal adenosis-adenocarcinoma [9,10]. A disturbed intrauterine *milieu interieur* brought on by endogenous factors, such carbohydrate intolerance, has further been shown to influence fetal growth and physiological adjustments predisposing the individual to adult-onset disease [11]; while exposure to nicotine from cigarette smoke has been shown to influence fetal growth and poor child neurodevelopment [12].

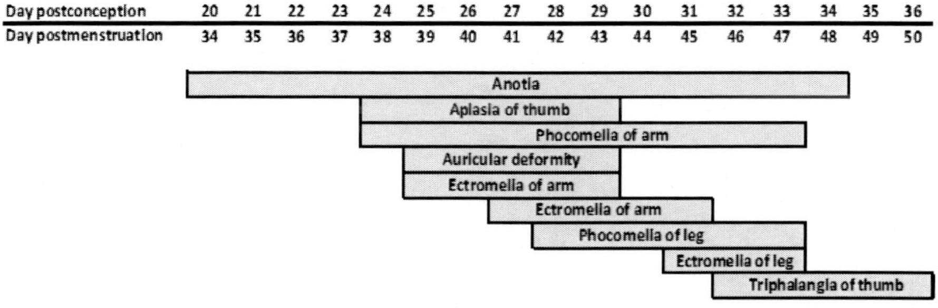

Figure 2. Teratogenic effects of thalidomide ingestion [7].

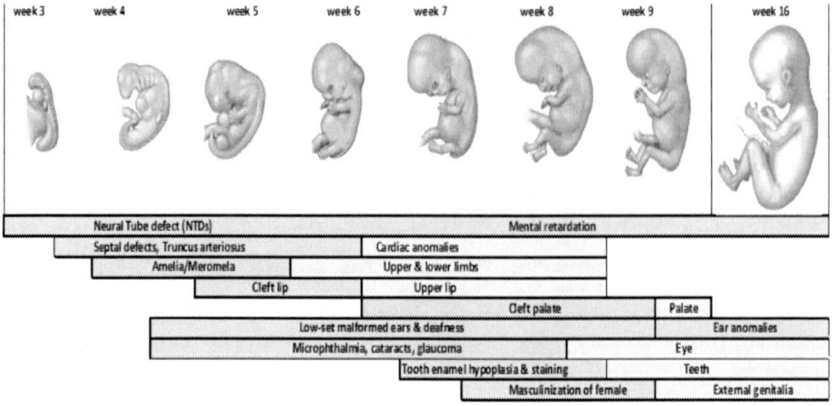

Figure 3. Embryogenesis.

Placental Transfer Mechanisms

The placenta starts to function from the fifth week onwards. The placenta is a complex organ that controls the passage of substances, including teratotoxic ones, from the mother to the developing embryo; and serves also as a metabolic organ having the capacity of altering the chemical structure of noxious substances making these less innocuous or alternatively more toxic. The passage of substances through the placenta does not solely depend on the process of simple diffusion, but also in some instances utilize active or facilitated transport mechanisms. Transfer of substances is thus dependent on the lipid or water solubility properties of the substance, the size of the molecule or whether it is protein or cell-bound, the degree of polarity or ionization and the pH of the substance. It also is dependent on the concentration and the degree of metabolism it undergoes within the syncyotiotrophoblast placental cells (Figure 4). The rate of transfer is dependent also on uterine blood flow which account for ~15% of cardiac output. Other potential mechanisms of placental transfer is by pinocytosis [e.g., immunoglobulins], and through breaks between the vascular compartments allowing transfer of placental or fetal cells [e.g., rhesus isoimmunization] to mother and maternal cells [e.g., melanoma or leukemic cells] to the fetus.

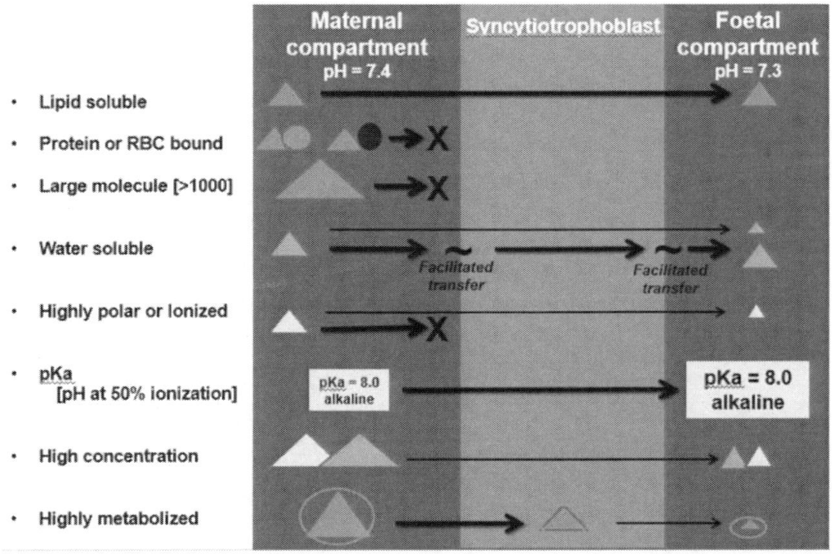

Figure 4. Placental transfer variables.

PHARMACOKINETICS OF TERATOLOGY

In pharmacology, any substance can be toxic if taken in a high enough dose with the efficacy-toxicity line being dependent on variables that are in play in the individual. All patented medications have a defined minimum effective dose [MED] and maximum tolerated dose [MTD]. The ideal pharmaceutical agent is one that has a large therapeutic window with a wide MED-MTD discrepancy. The narrow the discrepancy, the less safe is the agent for general use. The effective dose [ED_{50}] refers to the dose required to produce a desired therapeutic response in 50 percent of subjects. Similar pharmacokinetic principles can be applied to toxic agents. In 1927, the British pharmacologist J. W. Trevan in 1927 introduced the term "median lethal dose" or LD_{50} to refer to the dose that is needed to kill 50 percent of subjects. The LD_{50} value determines the sphere of action of a toxic substance into three zones: a non-lethal zone determined by the maximum tolerated safe dose; a zone of biological probability as determined by the LD_0 and LD_{100} where the effect of the agent on the organism is variable; and the lethal zone LD_{100} where all organisms are expected to die. The lower the LD_{50} value, the greater is the toxicity of the agent [13]. The LD_{50} values are different for different agents (Table 1) and will vary according to various factors including the species and mode of administration. In 1931, Kraber proposed a mathematical formula to calculate the LD_{50} using dose-related mortality rates under experimental conditions. Other modifications have since been proposed to Kraber's mathematical formula [14].

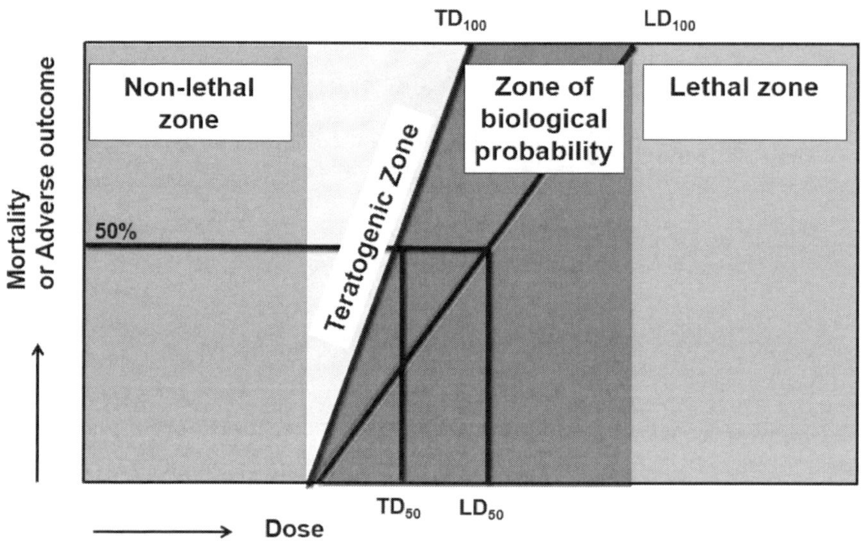

Figure 5. Fetal dose response chart.

Of course, the administration of a toxic substance has variable adverse outcomes other than death of the organism. Specific organ damage can occur without immediate death and hence the median lethal dose concept has to be tempered with considerations relating to "median adverse outcome dose" or AOD_{50} which is necessarily a different value to that of the LD_{50} for the same agent. The AOD_{50} is considered equivalent to the ratio of the dose necessary to cause 100 percent organ damage and that necessary to cause 100 percent mortality – AOD/LD_{100}. The adverse outcome principle can be extended to teratogenic damage of the developing fetus with teratotoxicity being dependent on the "median teratogenic dose" or TD_{50} which is similarly also equivalent to the TD/LD_{100}. In this scenario, the sphere of action of a toxic substance on the developing fetus now extends into four zones: a non-lethal zone; an adverse outcome or teratogenic zone; a zone of biological probability; and the lethal zone (Figure 5). This sphere of action must be tempered by considering also the toxic effect the agent has on the pregnant mother which similarly falls within the four zones but with different, generally higher, AOD_{50} and LD_{50} values.

VARIABLES AFFECTING TERATOGENIC DOSES

The median teratogenic dose is not a constant variable for all teratotoxic agents but is dependent of a number of variables that makes extrapolations from animal studies to humans difficult. There is also very little correlation between the maternal-LD_{50} and the fetal-TD/LD_{100} within the same species and the maternal-LD_{50}/fetal-TD/LD_{100} correlation ratio is different for different embryotoxic substances (Table 1) [15]. This is particularly evident for the antimetabolites tested where the correlation ratio ranges from 8 for 5-Fluorouracil to 50 for 6-Mercaptopurine riboside. Minor changes to the chemical formula can also result in significant changes in the correlation ratio: the ratio for 6-Mercaptopurine was 10, a figure that is in marked contrast to that of 6-Mercaptopurine riboside.

There is also very little correlation between the Fetal-TD/LD_{100} values for a particular teratotoxic agent in different animal species so that toxicology studies in animals cannot be transposed to humans. The classical studies on thalidomide demonstrated that there was a wide variation between different animal species in the lowest dose required to produce a teratogenic effect [16]. The teratogenic doses varies from 0.5-1.0 mg/kg/day in humans to as much as 350 mg/kg/day in the hamster (Table 2).

Table 1. Maternal LD50 and Fetal TD/LD100 in rat for various substances [15]

Agent	Maternal LD_{50} mg/kg	Fetal TD/LD_{100} mg/kg	Correlation ratio
Antibiotics			
Actinomycin D	0.4	0.3	1.3
Mitomycin	3.0	3.0	1
Streponigrin	0.4	0.2	2
Antimetabolites			
Azaserine	100	3	33
6-Mercaptopurine	250	25	10
6-Mercaptopurine	2000-3000	50	50
riboside	350	12	29
Thioguanine	200-400	15	20
Thioguanine riboside	230	30	8
5-Fluorouracil	17	0.5	34
Methotexate			
Alkylating agents			
Cyclophosphamide	40	15	3
Cholrambucil	24	6	4
Busulphan	60	18	3

Table 2. Lowest teratogenic dose for thalidomide by species [16]

Species	Lowest teratogenic dose Mg/kg/day
• Human	0.5-1.0
• Monkey	10
• Rabbit	30
• Mouse	31
• Rat	50
• Dog	100
• Hamster	350

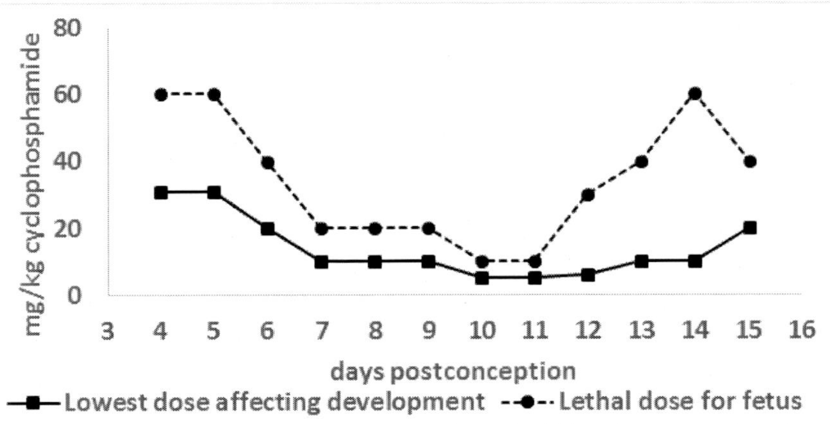

Figure 6. Teratotoxicity of cyclophosphamide in rat by gestational age [18].

The effective dose necessary to cause teratogenic effects for the same teratogen in a specific species also varies throughout gestation making predictions of teratotoxic effects of particular substances difficult with prolonged use. Cyclophosphamide is a widely used anticancer drug used also for its potent immunosuppressive properties in the management of systemic lupus erythematosus, rheumatoid arthritis, and nephrotic syndrome in childhood. The literature provides strong links between cyclophosphamide and a wide spectrum of teratogenic embryopathy particularly if the drug was administered during the first trimester of pregnancy [17]. The wide spectrum of abnormalities noted with cyclophosphamide use is in part dependent on the reported varying teratogenic dose susceptibility demonstrated during the first trimester use in the rat model (Figure 6) [18]. The teratotoxic effect of cyclophosphamide has also been shown to be reduced by the conjoint administration of folic acid, vitamin A and vitamin E [19].

Furthermore, the effect of a potential teratotoxic agent is sometimes mediated by the presence of a number of factors that range from the genetic makeup of the individual to the presence or absence of player substances. This is best exemplified by the teratotoxic effects of excessive Vitamin A ingestion. Vitamin A excess alone increases the risk of fetal anomalies characterized by anencephaly and cleft palate. The effect of

Vitamin A is potentiated by the administration of dexamethasone with thus serves to decrease the TD/LD_{100} of Vitamin A. In contrast, the conjoint administration of Vitamin B appears to be protective serving to increase the TD/LD_{100} of Vitamin A [20]. Genetic predispositions may also contribute towards enhancing the teratogenic effects of administered drugs. Acetaminophen used in the first trimester of pregnancy is associated with a risk of developing gastroschisis. Studies have suggested a link between gastroschisis development and the genetic variation in SULT1A3/4 in the human species [21]. Studies in humans relating specific genetic syndromes causing characteristic features with similar characteristic drug-induced embryopathies have indicated potential genetic phenocopies with embryopathies reported with use of thalidomide, warfarin, ACE inhibitors, fluconazole, leflunomide, mycophenolate, and mofetil. It appears that the phenocopies are caused be mutation of genes that encode the main target for the teratotoxin [22].

Mechanisms Driving Teratogenesis

Teratotoxic agents may exert their effects on directly on the developing cell at the cellular level influencing the intracellular compartment or the cell surface function. In the intracellular compartment, the teratogen directly or indirectly through its metabolic products influences the function of specific parts of the genetic code acting as inhibitors or stimulators. These effects would generally mimic and drive the development of phenocopies of specific genetic hereditary disorders. The cell surface in the developing zygote has important functions related to cell recognition and aggregation, intercellular interactions, and cellular migrations. Teratotoxic agents may again directly or indirectly influence cell surface structure and function (Figure 6). These processes would therefore potentially influence cellular reproduction, drive cellular death, and interfere with cellular organization or cellular migration [23]. The molecular cellular-driven teratogenesis includes epigenetic development caused by post-translational modifications of histone and DNA methylation driven by oxidative stress altering the metabolic pathways associated with methylation reaction [24].

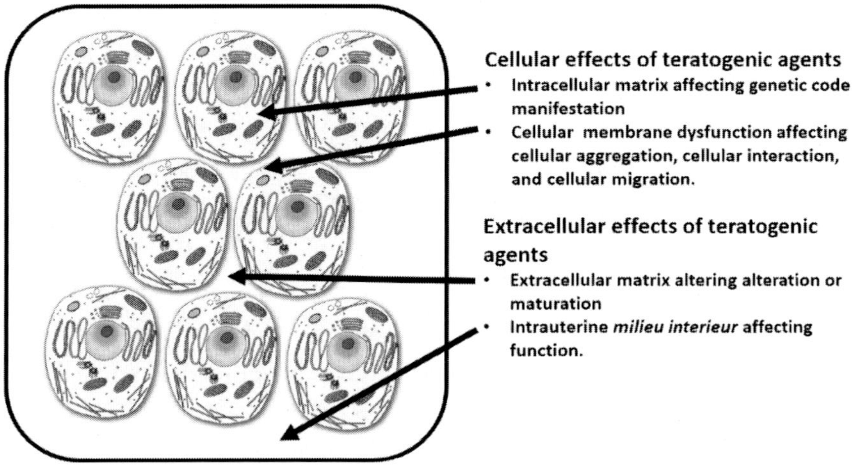

Figure 7. Teratogenic mechanisms of action.

The effect of the teratogen may also be exhibited directly or indirectly on the extracellular matrix or the overall *milieu interieur* of the developing zygote. The presence of the teratotoxic substance may thus interfere with the normal production or maturation of the extracellular matrix thus altering it sufficiently to drive abnormal development; while alterations in the *milieu interieur* could drive abnormalities at an organizational level or in the feto-maternal regulation by affecting hormonal and nutritional factors [23].

Discussion

The fetus developing in utero may be exposed to exogenous chemicals for a variety of reasons. These may directly or indirectly cause harm affecting its development. Medications in the first trimester of pregnancy may be partaken in the management of a chronic medical condition requiring regular treatment existing before the onset of cyesis. It is strongly recommended that pregnancies in women receiving any form of medication for a chronic medical condition should be planned and the medication reviewed in respect to its teratotoxic potential and changed accordingly. This preconceptional review is also particularly important in conditions that alter significantly the biochemical and hormonal *millieur interieur* of the mother and thus also of the developing fetus. This is strongly recommended in the situation where the mother suffers from diabetes mellitus where it has been shown that a poorly controlled carbohydrate metabolism state will in itself act as a teratotoxic agent increasing significantly the risk of fetal damage. In this situation, strict metabolic control has been in experimental and epidemiologic studies shown to reduce the incidence of birth defects. However, because many pregnancies are unplanned, preconceptional care is not regularly attested to even in the well-developed world [25]. Preconceptional care is also an opportunity to promote the use of folic acid supplementation at a dose of 0.4-1.0 mg daily which has been proven to decrease or minimize specific birth defects, particularly neural tube defects [NTD]. Women known to be at intermediate-high risk for neural tube defects should be prescribed higher folic acid doses of 4.0-5.0 mg daily provided these women have been shown not to suffer from Vitamin B12 deficiency. Women at high risk of neural tube defects include those with a family or personal previous history of a NTD-pregnancy, insulin-dependent diabetes, and those women receiving medication that has is a folate antagonist such as anti-epileptic medication e.g., valproic acid or carbamazepine [26]. Combined polypharmacy should be avoided. Multivitamin preparation formulations, especially those directed at general use, may include a significant dose of Vitamin A that itself alone can act as a teratotoxic agent on the fetus [20]. Preconceptional advice should also include advice about nutrition with an emphasis on partaking food items with a high antioxidant content to decrease the effect of oxidative stress known to act as a teratotoxic agent [27, 28].

Medications in the first trimester of pregnancy may be partaken to support the pregnancy or to manage a condition or distressing symptomatology that crops up during the pregnancy. The increasing use of reproductive technology has introduced an element of medicalization of pregnancy with attempts to support the early pregnancy state, a process that has extended to the management of recurrent pregnancy loss. These women are very often managed empirically using a combination of anticoagulation, progesterone supplementation, and immunomodulatory treatments [29, 30]. Such prescriptions must be tempered with an awareness of the potential teratotoxicity that this polypharmacy may contribute to and the knowledge that teratotoxicity may demonstrate itself in later years. One must bear in mind the past experience of the antenatal use of diethylstilboestrol in the management of miscarriages and the eventual development of vaginal adenosis-adenocarcinoma in the offspring [9, 10]. The thalidomide experience resulting from an attempt to manage the "normal" nausea and vomiting of pregnancy must also temper any attempts at managing non-life threatening symptomatology during early pregnancy. Any medications used during pregnancy should be restricted to those formulations that experience has shown to be non-teratotoxic and these should be used in isolation and for the shortest period of time and in the lowest dose possible. In the words of the seventeenth century English philosopher Sir Thomas Brown [*Religio Medici*; 1642]:

> "Every man is some months elder than he bethinks him; for we live, move, have a being and are subject to the actions of the elements and the malice of disease in that other World, the truest Microcosm, the Womb of our Mother."

References

[1] McBride W. G. Thalidomide and congenital abnormalities. *Lancet,* 1961; 2: 1358.

[2] Hardy J. B., McCracken G. H., Gilkeson M. R., Sever J. L. Adverse fetal outcome following maternal rubella after the first trimester of pregnancy. *JAMA,* 1969; 207(3): 2414-2420.

[3] Martin K. L. Nutritional and metabolic requirements of early cleavage stage embryos and blastocysts. *Hum Fertil*, 2000; 3(4): 247-254.

[4] Chico A., Herranz L., Corcoy R., Ramírez O., Goya M. M., Bellart J., González-Romero S., Codina M., Sánchez P., Cortázar A., Acosta D., Picón M. J., Rubio J. A., Megía A., Sancho M. A., Balsells M., Solá E., González NL, López-López J; GEDE (Group of Diabetes and Pregnancy of the Spanish Diabetes Association). Glycemic control and maternal and fetal outcomes in pregnant women with type 1 diabetes according to the type of basal insulin. *Eur J Obstet Gynecol Reprod Biol,* 2016 Nov; 206: 84-91.

[5] Eckert J. J., Fleming T. P. The effect of nutrition and environment on the preimplantation embryo. *Obstetrician Gynaecologist*, 2011, 13: 43-48.

[6] Vargesson N. Thalidomide-induced teratogenesis: History and mechanisms. *Birth Defects Res C Embryo Today*, 2015; 105(2): 140–156.

[7] Nowack E. The sensitive phase in thalidomide embryopathy. *Humangenetik,* 1965; 1:516–536.

[8] Gales D., Hewitt D., Stewart A., Webb J. Malignant disease in childhood and diagnostic irradiation in utero. *Lancet,* 1956; 271(6940): 447.

[9] Herbst A. L., Ulfelder H., Poskanzer D. C. Adenocarcinoma of the vagina. Association of stilbestrol therapy with tumor appearance in young women. *New Engl J Med*, 1971; 284: 878-881.

[10] Herbst A. L., Norusis M. J., Rosenow P. J., Welch W. R., Scully R. E. An analysis of 346 cases of clear cell carcinoma of the vagina and cervix with emphasis on recurrence and survival. *Gynecol Obstet*, 1979; 7: 111-122.

[11] Aerts L., Van Assche A. Is gestational diabetes an acquired condition? *J Developmental Physiology*, 1979; 1: 219-225.

[12] Polańska K., Jurewicz J., Hanke W. Smoking and alcohol drinking during pregnancy as the risk factors for poor child neurodevelopment

- A review of epidemiological studies. *Int J Occup Med Environ Health.* 2015; 28(3): 419-443.

[13] Trevan J. W. The Error of Determination of Toxicity. *Proc Roy Soc* B, 1927; 101(712): 483-514.

[14] Chinedu E., Arome D., Ameh F. S. A New Method for Determining Acute Toxicity in Animal Models. *Toxicol Int*, 2013; 20(3): 224–226.

[15] Murphy M. L. Teratogenic effects in rats of growth inhibiting chemicals, including studies on thalidomide. *Clin Proc Child Hosp Dist Columbia*, 1962; 18: 307-322.

[16] McColl J. D. Drug toxicity in the animal fetus. *Appl Ther*, 1967; 9(11): 915-917.

[17] Rengasamy P. 1. Congenital Malformations Attributed to Prenatal Exposure to Cyclophosphamide. *Anticancer Agents Med Chem.* 2016 Dec 6, 16: E-pub Ahead of Print.

[18] Kreybig T. Die teratogene Wirkung von Cyclophosphamid während der embryonalen Entwicklungsphase bei der Ratte. *Naunyn-Schmiedebergs Arch Pharmak exp Path*, 1965; 252: 172–195.

[19] Ma A., Xu H., Du W., Liu Y. Effect of folic acid and supplemented with vitamin A and vitamin E on depressing teratogenesis induced by cyclophosphamide. *Wei Sheng Yan Jiu,* 2001; 30(6): 343-346.

[20] Natsume N., Narukawa T., Kawai T. Teratogenesis of dexamethasone and preventive effect of vitamin B12. *Inter J Oral Maxilofacial Surg,* 1986, 15(6): 752-755.

[21] Adjei A. A., Gaedigk A., Simon S. D., Weinshilboum R. M., Leeder J. S. Interindividual variability in acetaminophen sulfation by human fetal liver: implications for pharmacogenetic investigations of drug-induced birth defects. *Birth Defects Res A Clin Mol Teratol*, 2008; 2(3): 155-665.

[22] Cassina M., Cagnoli G. A., Zuccarello D., Di Gianantonio E., Clementi M. Human teratogens and genetic phenocopies. Understanding pathogenesis through human genes mutation. *Eur J Med Genet*, 2017; 60(1): 22-31.

[23] Saxen L. Mechanisms of teratogenesis. *J Embryol exp Morph*, 1976; 36(1): 1-12.

[24] Nagai K. Epigenetic developmental origins hypothesis and oxidative stress. In: Matata BM, Maqsood MM [editors]. *The Molecular Basis for the link between maternal health and the origin of fetal congenital abnormalities – An overview of association with oxidative stress.* USA, Bentham, 2011; 50-57.

[25] Reece E. A. Diabetes-induced birth defects: what do we know? What can we do? *Curr Diab Rep*, 2012; 12(1): 24-32.

[26] Wilson R. D., Davies G., Désilets V., Reid G. J., Summers A., Wyatt P., Young D., Genetics Committee and Executive and Council of the Society of Obstetricians and Gynaecologists of Canada. The use of folic acid for the prevention of neural tube defects and other congenital anomalies. *J Obstet Gynaecol Can*, 2003; 25(11): 959-973.

[27] Cederberg J., Simán C. M., Eriksson U. J. Combined treatment with vitamin E and vitamin C decreases oxidative stress and improves fetal outcome in experimental diabetic pregnancy. *Pediatr Res*, 2001; 49(6):755-762.

[28] Ornoy A. Embryonic oxidative stress as a mechanism of teratogenesis with special emphasis on diabetic embryopathy. *Reprod Toxicol,* 2007; 24(1): 31-41.

[29] El Hachem H., Crepaux V., May-Panloup P., Descamps P., Legendre G., Bouet P. E. Recurrent pregnancy loss: current perspectives. *Int J Womens Health,* 2017; 9: 331-345.

[30] Sugiura-Ogasawara M., Ozaki Y., Suzumori N. Management of recurrent miscarriage. *J Obstet Gynaecol Res*, 2014; 40(5): 1174-1179.

In: An Essential Guide … ISBN: 978-1-53613-331-8
Editors: A. Goodwin and S. Lynch

Chapter 7

PERCEPTIONS OF MOTIVES FOR CONTRACEPTIVE INTERFERENCE: PATTERNS OF GENDER DIFFERENCE AND SIMILARITY

Jennifer Katz, Jillian LaRose and Brittney Richardson
State University of New York at Geneseo, NY, US

ABSTRACT

Contraceptive interference (CI) occurs when a person directly interferes with his or her partner's ability to effectively use contraception before or during sex. Perceived motives for CI warrant empirical study. We hypothesized that common barriers to male condom use might also be perceived as motives for CI enacted by a man toward his female partner. In addition, we explored potential gender differences in perceptions of these motives. Undergraduates with prior vaginal sex experience (N = 334) read a hypothetical vaginal sex scenario depicting a man's CI behavior. Then participants rated the degree to which they perceived different barriers to male condom use may have motivated the man's behavior. Results showed that all participants perceived that a man's CI behavior was motivated by his intent to enhance his pleasure. Compared to women, men more strongly perceived a man's CI behaviors occurred because the female partner was using another type of birth control, to promote female pleasure, and because the man preferred not to discuss condoms. Compared to men, women more strongly perceived a man's CI behaviors occurred because the female partner was faithful and because the man felt using condoms was difficult. These results suggest that interventions geared toward preventing CI should emphasize that even behaviors apparently motivated by benign intent may yield negative sexual and reproductive health consequences.

INTRODUCTION

Reproductive coercion (RC) involves acts of "power and control in a relationship related to reproductive health" (Chamberlain & Levenson, 2016, p. 6) that increase risk for adverse outcomes such as unintended pregnancy and STIs (Kazmerski et al., 2015). RC behaviors, which are related to behaviors that affect contraceptive use and pregnancy outcomes, tend to be enacted by men towards women within heterosexual relationships. In early studies, RC was operationally defined as behaviors perceived as intending to promote pregnancy or control pregnancy outcomes (Miller at al., 2010). The central role of perceived intent is highlighted in the definition of RC provided by Moore, Frohwirth, and Miller (2010), who wrote that RC "occurs when women's partners demand or enforce their own reproductive intentions" (p. 1738). The most widely used operational definitions of reproductive coercion assess both *pregnancy coercion,* pressure to get pregnant or not to use birth control, and *birth control sabotage*, acts of direct contraceptive interference perceived to be motivated by the partner's intent to promote pregnancy (Chamberlain & Levenson, 2016; Miller et al., 2010).

CI is very similar to, and a critical component of, birth control sabotage. Unlike birth control sabotage, however, contraceptive interference is defined solely in terms of behavior, regardless of the perceived intent. That is, a woman who experiences CI may not necessarily perceive her partner's CI behaviors were motivated by an intent to promote pregnancy. For example, in a study of sexually active college women, 21% reported that a male partner made them have sex without a condom and/or removed a condom during sex without their knowledge or consent (Katz, Poleshuck, Beach, & Olin, 2017). Other examples of contraceptive interference (CI) include taking condoms or other birth control away or tearing a condom on purpose.

Restricting conceptual and operational definitions of RC, and specifically, birth control sabotage, to acts perceived as intended to promote or control pregnancy appears to underestimate how many women are constrained in protecting their reproductive and sexual health. In a recent study of sexually active college women, Katz and Sutherland (2017) found that 25% reported lifetime CI experiences. When asked about their perceptions of reasons for this behavior, all of these women perceived that partners had interfered with contraception to enhance their own pleasure. Most also perceived that partners felt using condoms was difficult and ruined the mood. Other commonly endorsed perceived reasons included the partner's knowledge that she was using other methods of birth control, the partner's trust that she was monogamous, the partner's interest in feeling closer to one another, and the partner's interest in enhancing the woman's pleasure. Very few women perceived that their past partner enacted CI to promote pregnancy (8%, n = 3). Furthermore, no women strongly agreed with these perceptions; rather, one respondent slightly agreed with this statement, and two respondents somewhat agreed. These findings suggest that women with actual experiences of CI rarely perceived that such experiences were based on the partner's interest in promoting pregnancy.

To our knowledge, no studies have examined men's reports of reasons for enacting CI. In addition, no studies have examined whether women and men show similar or divergent perceptions of reasons for enacting CI behavior. Given that past research has shown gender differences in attitudes about male condom use (e.g., East, Jackson, O'Brien, & Peters, 2007), and given that CI seems to frequently involve interfering with condoms, it seems likely that there may also be gender differences in perceptions of reasons for contraceptive interference. Barriers to male condom use, which include beliefs that condoms reduce intimacy and pleasure for both partners (e.g., Geter & Crosby, 2014) might also be factors perceived to underlie condom-related contraceptive interference. Accordingly, the current study explored perceptions of reasons for contraceptive interference involving a heterosexual couple in which the male partner removes the condom without his female partner's knowledge or consent. We sought to identify perceptions of common reasons for CI among both women and men as well as potential gender differences in these perceptions.

METHOD

Participants

Undergraduate students (N = 334) were eligible for this study if they had been previously involved in a sexual relationship involving vaginal intercourse. More women (77.2%) than men (22.8%) participated. Most were freshmen (34.9%) or sophomores (36.4%) although some juniors (17.8%) and seniors (10.8%) were also represented. Participants' average age was 19.24 (SD = 1.26, range 17 to 28). Most participants self-identified as White (81.1%); others identified as Asian or Asian-American (8.7%), Hispanic/Latina (4.2%), Black or African-American (3.6%), or "other" (2.4%).

Measures

In response to a scenario in which the male partner interferes with effective contraceptive use during sex with a female partner, participants were asked to rate to what extent they thought the male partner's behavior was motivated by each of 12 factors. These factors were based on the motives studied by Katz and Sutherland (2017), who conducted a literature review of barriers to male condom use. These barriers included concerns about condoms decreasing male pleasure (e.g., Crosby, Charnigo, & Shrier, 2014; Geter & Crosby, 2014; Moore & Halford, 1999; Sakar, 2008) as well as female partner pleasure or enjoyment (Geter & Crosby, 2014). Other barriers to condom use included creating potential lack of intimacy (Geter & Crosby, 2014) and perceiving that relationship commitment/ monogamy justifies not using condoms (e.g., Sakar, 2008). Condoms also may be perceived as difficult to talk about (Moore & Halford, 1999; Widman, Noar, Choukas-Bradley, & Francis, 2014), prohibited by one's religious tradition (Sakar, 2008), avoided due to alcohol or drug use (Brafford & Beck, 1991; Tubman, Langer, & Shams, 2003) or inconsistent with perceived social norms (Geter & Crosby, 2014). Specific items for barriers to condom use that were studied as potential motives for contraceptive interference are listed in Table 1. Possible responses to each item were rated on a 4 point scale (1 = *not at all*, 4 = *very much*).

Procedure

Participants were recruited for a study of "Condom Use Behaviors, Attitudes, and Conflict" through a voluntary psychology department pool. Data were collected in single research sessions lasting no more than one hour. Research sessions were administered in small groups in campus classrooms by a trained female undergraduate. All participants provided informed consent and completed self-report paper and pencil measures regarding their past experiences with vaginal sex. They also responded to their perceptions about the male partner's behavior in the following scenario:

> "Nate and Holly have been dating for close to a year. They generally always use condoms, and the last time they had sex was no different. During sex, though, Nate removed the condom without telling Holly, so they ended up having sex without a condom. If you had to guess, to what extent to do you think Nate's actions were because he…."

All participants were offered extra credit for their time, were fully debriefed, and provided with information about healthy and destructive conflict within intimate relationships. All study materials and procedures were approved by the campus Institutional Review Board.

Table 1. Gender Differences in Perceptions of Reasons for Contraceptive Interference

Motive	Overall	Women (n = 248)	Men (n = 71)	$F(1, 317)$
wanted to make sex feel better for him	3.78 (0.50)	3.81 (0.44)	3.67 (0.69)	3.87*
felt using condoms was difficult/a hassle	2.99 (1.02)	3.08 (1.00)	2.68 (1.05)	8.69**
trusted she was faithful	2.69 (1.00)	2.63 (1.02)	2.46 (0.99)	3.67*
knew she was using other birth control	2.60 (0.94)	2.52 (9.94)	2.87 (0.87)	7.91**
wanted them to feel closer to each other	2.49 (0.99)			1.70
wanted to make sex feel better for her	2.41 (0.97)	2.33 (0.97)	2.68 (0.95)	7.09**
didn't like having to talk about condoms	2.15 (0.99)	2.24 (0.99)	2.63 (0.99)	10.46***
his friends don't think condoms are important	2.00 (0.89)			1.36
was using alcohol or drugs	1.93 (0.87)			<1
didn't think condoms are effective	1.28 (0.62)			<1
wanted her to get pregnant	1.16 (0.45)			<1
had religious concerns about using condoms	1.09 (0.32)			<1

Notes: $^{*}p < .05$, $^{**}p < .01$, $^{***}p < .001$. Means and standard deviations are reported

RESULTS

A single factor (participant gender) between-subjects MANOVA was conducted with each of the 12 motives for contraceptive interference (CI) as the dependent measures. There was a significant main effect of participant gender, F (12, 306) = 2.75, p = .001, η^2 = .10, suggesting significant gender differences in perceived motives underlying CI. Univariate follow up analyses are reported in Table 1. Items are listed in descending mean order for the sample.

Gender differences emerged for the more common motives perceived to underlie a man's use of contraceptive interference behaviors. As can be seen, compared to men, women perceived increased male pleasure, male difficulties with condom use, and female faithfulness as stronger motives for a man's CI behaviors. Compared to women, men perceived the female partner's use of other forms of birth control, interest in female pleasure, and male avoidance of discussing condom use as stronger motives for a man's CI behaviors. There were no gender differences in perceptions of other motives.

CONCLUSION

The current study investigated the perceptions that both women and men have about why a man would enact contraceptive interference (CI) during a sexual interaction with his female partner. CI is a behaviorally specific version of birth control sabotage that, unlike birth control sabotage, is not necessarily perceived to be motivated by an intent to promote or control pregnancy. Overall, the most common perceived motives for contraceptive interference (CI) were related to promoting male pleasure, difficulties using condoms, trust in female faithfulness, and reliance on other forms of birth control. These perceptions of reasons for CI strongly converge with past research focused on women who have actually experienced CI. That is, the motives that participants most often endorsed as likely to explain a man's CI behaviors in the current study matched closely with the reasons that women most often endorsed as likely related to why a male partner had enacted CI (Katz & Sutherland, 2017).

Also as expected, gender differences emerged in the degree to which some motives were perceived as underlying CI behavior. Compared to men, women perceived increased male pleasure, male difficulties with condom use, and female faithfulness as stronger motives for contraceptive interference. Compared to women, men perceived partner use of other forms of birth control, interest in female pleasure, and male avoidance of discussing condom use as stronger motives for contraceptive interference. The current findings therefore expand past research on gender differences in attitudes about condom use (e.g., East et al., 2007) to show gender differences in perceptions of why male partners might sabotage condom use during sex.

Despite these gender differences, there was also evidence for similar perceptions of motives for CI across gender. Notably, the current results suggest both women and men alike perceived that interest in enhancing male pleasure was the most common motive underlying CI. This was also the most common perceived motive for CI reported by college women who actually experienced CI (Katz & Sutherland, 2017). Neither women nor men tended to perceive that CI was motivated by peer norms for condom use, alcohol or drug use, beliefs about condoms as ineffective, religious concerns, or interest in promoting pregnancy. Again, these same motives were infrequently cited by women with actual CI experiences (Katz & Sutherland, 2017). The current study, combined with past research, suggests that college students reliably perceive more and less common reasons for sabotaging contraceptive use during hetero(sex) both across gender and regardless of whether they have personally experienced or enacted CI.

The current results are limited by the reliance on a convenience sample of students reporting on a hypothetical scenario. It is unknown how many of these students have personal experiences with CI that may have informed their perceptions of the scenario. Future studies of gender differences in perceived motives for actual experiences of CI are a priority for future investigations. Studies involving dyads may reveal important relationship characteristics important in the assessment of CI and RC. In addition, studies of men who enact CI are needed, including studies of men's reported motives for enacting CI, factors that inhibit them from enacting such behaviors, and the role of psychoeducation in fostering prosocial attitudes about and avoidance of CI behaviors.

The current results add to a growing literature that challenges definitions of RC tying behaviors that sabotage effective contraceptive use to the perception of intent to promote pregnancy. College students infrequently perceived intent to promote pregnancy as a motive for CI, both in the current study and in past research focused on women with CI experiences (Katz & Sutherland, 2017). Given that past research suggests that between 20 and 25% of sexually active college women have experienced behaviorally specific CI enacted by a male partner (Katz et al., 2017), overly restrictive definitions fail to identify the majority of women who have experienced limited control over their own reproductive health.

In conclusion, the current results suggest that many women and men perceive that CI behaviors occur due to benign or even generous intent (e.g., to promote intimacy, as a sign of trust). These perceptions have important applied implications. More specifically, educational efforts aimed at preventing CI behaviors should acknowledge the full range of motives that may underlie such behaviors. Such educational efforts must also highlight the potential difference between positive intent and negative consequences for women's reproductive and sexual health.

REFERENCES

Brafford, L. J., & Beck, K. H. (1991). Development and validation of a condom self-efficacy scale for college students. *Journal of American College Health, 39*, 219-225.

Chamberlain, L., & Levenson, R. (2016). Addressing intimate partner violence, reproductive and sexual coercion: A guide for obstetric, gynecologic, and reproductive health care settings. 2nd Edition. *Family*

Violence Prevention Fund. Retrieved from http://www.community solutionsva.org/index.php/resources/item/addressing-intimate-partner-violence-reproductive-and-sexual-coercion-guide.

Crosby, R. A., Charnigo, R., & Shrier, L. A. (2014). Prospective associations between perceived barriers to condom use and "perfect use." *American Journal of Preventive Medicine, 47*, 70-72.

East, L., Jackson, D., O'Brien, L., & Peters, K. (2007). Use of the male condom by heterosexual adolescents and young people: Literature review. *Journal of Advanced Nursing, 59,* 103-110.

Geter, A., & Crosby, R. (2014). Condom refusal and young black men: The influence of pleasure, sexual partners, and friends. *Journal of Urban Health, 91*, 541-546.

Katz, J., Poleshuck, E., Beach, B., & Olin, R. (2017). Reproductive coercion by male sexual partners: Associations with partner violence and college women's sexual health. *Journal of Interpersonal Violence, 32,* 3301-3320. doi: 10.1177/0886260515597441.

Katz, J., & Sutherland, M. (2017). College women's experiences of male partner contraceptive interference: Associations with intimate partner violence and contraceptive outcomes. *Journal of Interpersonal Violence.* Advance online publication doi: 10.1177/088626051771 5600.

Kazmerski, T., McCauley, H. L., Jones, K., Borrero, S., Silverman, J. G., Decker, M. R., & Miller, E. (2014). Use of reproductive and sexual health services among female family planning clinic clients exposed to partner violence and reproductive coercion. *Maternal and Child Health Journal, 19,* 1490-1496.

Miller, E., Decker, M. R., McCauley, H. I., Tancredit, D. J., Levenson, R. R., Waldman, J. Schoenwald, P., & Silverman, J. G. (2010). Pregnancy coercion, intimate partner violence, and unintended pregnancy. *Contraception*, 81, 316-322.

Moore, S., & Halford, A. P. (1999). Barriers to safer sex: Beliefs and attitudes among male and female adult heterosexuals across four relationship groups. *Journal of Health Psychology, 4*, 149-163.

Sakar, N. N. (2008). Barriers to condom use. *The European Journal of Contraception and Reproductive Health Care*, *13*, 114-122.

Tubman, J. G., Langer, L. M., & Shams, S. (2003). Condom use, condom refusal, and substituted sexual behaviors among youth at higher and lower risk for HIV infection. *Journal of Social Work Practice in the Addictions*, *3*, 73-91.

Widman, L., Noar, S. M., Choukas-Bradley, S., & Francis, D. B. (2014). Adolescent sexual health communication and condom use: A meta-analysis. *Health Psychology, 33*, 1113-1124.

INDEX

A

B

C

D

E

N

O

P

Q

R

S

T

U

V

W

Y

Z